OLDER
ADULTS
IN
PSYCHOTHERAPY

Case Histories

OLDER
ADULTS
IN
PSYCHOTHERAPY

Case Histories

Bob G. Knight

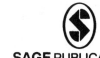

SAGE PUBLICATIONS
The International Professional Publishers
Newbury Park   London   New Delhi

For information address:

 SAGE Publications, Inc.
2455 Teller Road
Newbury Park, California 91320

SAGE Publications Ltd.
6 Bonhill Street
London EC2A 4PU
United Kingdom

SAGE Publications India Pvt. Ltd.
M-32 Market
Greater Kailash I
New Delhi 110 048 India

Printed in the United States of America

Library of Congress Cataloging-in-Publication Data

Knight, Bob G.
   Older adults in psychotherapy : case histories/ Bob G. Knight.
      p.   cm.
   ISBN 0-8039-3628-1.   —   ISBN 0-8039-3629-X (pbk.)
   1. Psychotherapy for the aged—Case studies. I. Title .
RC480.54.K65   1992
618.97'68914—dc20   19-37182

        94 95 10 9 8 7 6 5 4 3 2

Sage Production Editor: Diane S. Foster

Contents

Acknowledgments

It was Terry Hendrix, then my editor at Sage Publications, who first recognized the need for this book and talked me into writing it. For that, and for his patience as I prepared to do the writing, I am very grateful. Marquita Fleming, who took over as project editor, has been kind and encouraging at every stage of the development of this book.

A most heartfelt thanks to the 18 individuals who shared their lives with me as their therapist and were also willing to have those lives shared with others in this book. They have taught me much, first as clients and then by allowing the rethinking process of writing about them. I also gratefully acknowledge the scores of other clients whose experiences form the unseen backdrop for this book.

My professional career has been lived within two institutional environments: the Senior Outreach Services of Ventura County Mental Health Services and the Andrus Gerontology Center of the University of Southern California. The psychotherapists, administrators, faculty, and students in those settings have taught me a great deal and have forced me to reevaluate what I thought I knew.

Martha Storandt of Washington University provided the intial impetus and direction for a renewed study of gerontology and what it offers the psychotherapist. Sandra Powers of the University of North Carolina (Greensboro) has more than once helped me to understand that some of what was obvious to me about working with older adults is controversial to others.

Hortense Tingstad and Merle H. Bensinger have, in different ways, encouraged and supported my work at the Andrus Gerontology Center and have inspired my thinking about maturity and the courage to face life's challenges.

My mother Betty Foster has passed on to me her love of writing and her love of older people. My daughter Carmen is teaching me about the nature of development. My wife Patty has helped to keep me thinking clearly.

simplify the field and disagree with some persons in it. As in the first volume, my intent is to convey major concepts and findings from gerontology to psychotherapists—and to encourage therapists to read more of gerontology so they can stay current with a rapidly developing science and find answers to specific questions about older clients.

Intelligence and Memory in Late Life. The most pervasive cognitive change with developmental aging is the slowing of response that occurs in all tasks where speed of response is a factor (Botwinick, 1984; Salthouse, 1985). While reaction time can be speeded up in older adults by practice, exercise, and other interventions, the age difference is seldom completely eliminated. In a thorough review of this literature, Salthouse argues convincingly that the probable locus of slowing is in the central nervous system.

Intelligence can be divided up in a number of ways. In the study of aging, tasks that involve a speeded or timed component show clear evidence of change with developmental aging. The types of tasks most often associated with intelligence in adults, such as general fund of information, vocabulary, and arithmetic skills, show little change as a result of the aging process until age 75 or so (Schaie, 1983). Changes after 75 are largely unstudied and very difficult to untangle from changes in persons of advanced age that could be signs of Alzheimer's disease or other dementing illness in the early stages.

There are cohort differences in intellectual skills, however. In general, Schaie's Seattle study shows that later-born cohorts tend to be superior in reasoning ability. On the other hand, some earlier-born cohorts (people who are now older) are superior in arithmetic ability and verbal fluency. This examples illustrates the important point that the absence of developmental change does not necessarily mean that older people, as they exist today, are not different from today's younger people. This example also shows that some differences between cohorts favor the older cohort.

Rybash, Hoyer, and Roodin (1986) advance some intriguing notions about the course of cognitive development across the adult life span. Drawing on the information-processing "mind as computer" metaphor, they argue that increased experience can be seen as operating like an "expert system" program. With the accumulation of experience, older adults have a considerable store of knowledge about how things are and how things work, especially in their individual areas of expertise informed by work experience and family experiences. In these expert domains, the more mature may tend to outperform the young. In contrast, perhaps the excess speed and energy of the young are helpful in processing much new information without the aid of an expert system. In a somewhat related vein, Salthouse (1985) speculated that slowing with age could be due to older adults having developed a machine language (the internal control language of the "mind as computer"), which handles abstract material better and faster but at the cost of slowing down in the lower level tasks typically measured in reaction time experiments (e.g., speed of hitting a lever after hearing a tone).

Rybash et al. also argue for the existence of a postformal stage of cognitive development for more mature adults. Beyond the abstract thinking, deductive ability, and symbol manipulation of the formal stage, the postformal stage would include dialectical thinking, an appreciation of the truth of ideas depending on context, and the ability to hold two opposing viewpoints in mind at the same time. They acknowledge evidence that many adults have not reached the formal stage, and that both formal and postformal stages seem to be confounded with level of education. The notion is intriguing and consistent with clinical observation of greater complexity of thinking in older clients.

Memory is perhaps the most difficult topic in the study of cognitive changes in late life. In sharp contrast to the methodological sophistication of studies of intellectual change in aging, most memory studies are cross-sectional, and so compare older adults with younger adults at one point in time, confounding aging effects and cohort differences. Longitudinal studies with the Wechsler Memory Scale show little developmental change in memory when health is statistically controlled (Siegler, 1983). Reisberg, Shulman, Ferris, de Leon, and Geibel (1983) have identified older adults with memory problems and followed them over time. They report that most older adults with memory changes, even changes that interfere with complex work or social activities, do not develop progressive memory loss. While there are clearly increasing numbers of dementing older adults with each decade of advanced age, it is unclear whether there are also benign memory changes in normal aging. The problem is methodologically challenging and has important implications for both our understanding of normal aging and our ability to estimate the prevalence of disorders like Alzheimer's disease in very late life.

In general, what is known about memory now would suggest that even differences between current younger and older adults in memory performance are not large when the material is meaningful and relevant to the older adult, and the older adult is motivated to learn (Botwinick, 1984; Craik & Trehub, 1982; L. Light, 1990; Poon, 1985). In contrast, younger adults do better on novel information and learning tasks with no intrinsic meaning (learning a list of nonsense words, for example). One aspect of relevance of materials is the discovery that older adults learn word lists better when the lists are made of "old words" (e.g., *fedora*) as opposed to "new words." This finding demonstrates that word usage changes over time and suggests that therapists need to consider using appropriate word choices when communicating with older adults.

An intriguing problem in this area is that older adults do not spontaneously use mnemonic aids. They can be taught to do so and will improve their memory performance substantially. However, they have to be reminded to use the mnemonic aids at the next session (cf. Botwinick, 1984). If this tendency to need prompting to use newly learned strategies generalizes to the therapeutic context, it would be important even if specific to current cohorts of the elderly.

In applying these findings to the need to change therapy when working with older adults, the following general conclusions can be argued. For healthy older adults, there is no reason to alter the work of therapy based on normal developmental changes that occur with aging, at least until about 75 to 80 years of age. As I suggested in the earlier book, the pace of conversation may be slower with older adults, but the overall speed of therapy in terms of number of sessions does not change up until this age range. In fact, in two studies I have shown that older adults progress more in therapy than do younger adults, as measured by therapist ratings of change (Knight, 1983, 1988). In the second study (Knight,

1988), there appeared to be a need for more sessions of therapy with the old-old (80+) to achieve change equivalent to what was obtained with young-old (60-69) clients in brief therapy.

There are two important qualifications to this general conclusion that psychotherapy need not be limited by developmental changes in intelligence and memory. First, older people are more often suffering from disease, especially from chronic illness or disability. Most systemic disease in late life will produce additional slowing in reaction time and in the pace of speech and comprehension. Working with the ill elderly will likely require both a conscious effort to slow the pace of conversation and a greater number of therapeutic visits for equivalent therapeutic change.

The second qualification is that these observations are based on the absence of *developmental* change. There are cohort differences in intellectual abilities and level of education. As is true in work with younger adults, the client's level of education, vocabulary, familiarity with psychological terms, and ability to engage in abstract thinking must be taken into account. In general, these changes would be similar in kind to adapting therapy to working with lower SES clients (cf. Goldstein, 1973; Lorion, 1978). While this is a cohort difference rather than an aging issue, it is not trivial in thinking about adapting therapy to work with older adults, or in educating therapists about working with the elderly. It may be necessary to use less psychological jargon, to use more concrete examples, and to use more repetition. These adaptations are based on the historical fact of earlier cohorts having less education, less exposure to psychological concepts, and so forth. Understanding the adaptations to be due to these other cohort-based differences rather than to aging has the advantage of being accurate, of guiding the practitioner to other literature on adaptation of therapy, and of not overgeneralizing the need to adapt: That is, there are older people with statistically atypical backgrounds who will be very ready for therapy. Some of the case histories in this volume are about such older clients.

The work by Rybash et al. (1986), exploring the possibility of greater cognitive complexity in more mature adults and calling attention to the role of experience-based expertise, points to some cognitive strengths that older adults bring to therapy. Virtually all of the older clients I have seen know more about some areas of life than I do. Especially relevant to the therapeutic enterprise is the background of a lifetime of experience in relationships and the experience of playing differing roles in relationships. Whereas clients in early adulthood are entering adult life with experience of their family of origin, some school friendships, and some experience of love, older adults have been children, parents, grandparents, siblings; have had many friendships, lovers, and work relationships. In addition to personal experience, most people have considerable vicarious experience watching what happens to friends, family, and colleagues in relationships and in life more generally. These experiences have led to the distillation of concepts about how life and relationships work, a kind of psychological "expert system." Much of this system may be accurate; some may need to be challenged and reworked. In either case, it represents a wealth of ideas and strengths that older people bring to therapy. Much of therapy with young adults seems to involve encouraging them to explore unknown potential in their lives. Much of therapy with older adults involves encouraging the rediscovery and use of known skills and expertise.

Personality and Emotional Development. There is much more available research on personality development in adulthood and later life than there was 5 years ago. The work of Costa, McCrae, and associates in the Baltimore Longitudinal Study on Aging (McCrae & Costa, 1984), using self-report measures of personality and a nomothetic model of personality measurement, has supported stability of personality across the adult life span with the greatest certainty of stability from age 30 to age 60. Their sample is mostly male and middle-class to upper middle-class. The dimensions on which they find stability include introversion/extroversion, neuroticism, openness to experience, dependability, and agreeableness. These results are not trivial; they argue strongly against the Jungian notion that late life involves a switch to polar opposites on traits to achieve a balanced personality (Jung, 1933). They also argue against common notions of older adults withdrawing socially or becoming less interested in new experiences. Based on their data, Costa and McCrae (1985) have argued against the concept that older adults become more hypochondriacal and against a normative mid-life crisis. They also find cohort effects in personality; for example, later-born cohorts are less restrained and higher in dominance than persons born earlier in this century (Costa, McCrae, & Arenberg, 1983). In general, their results argue that observed personality differences between young people and older adults are more likely to be cohort differences than those due to aging as a developmental process.

Using a very different methodology that included interviewer ratings rather than self-report and an ipsative model of personality that leads to description of the relative salience of dimensions within the individual rather than the person's ranking in the group on predetermined scales, Haan, Millsap, and Hartka (1986) reported on the Oakland Guidance study of both men and women from age 7 to about age 60. They found stability for cognitive commitment, dependability, and outgoingness, dimensions that are conceptually similar to openness to experience, dependability, and introversion-extroversion in the Costa et al. studies. They found self-confident/victimized (similar to neuroticism) to be stable across the adult years for men but not for women. In general, they found women to be more flexible in organization of personality across the life span than were men. They conclude that in spite of considerable stability across many transitions, the organization of personality in late life is very different from that of childhood. They found childhood to early adolescence to be the most stable period of life, followed by considerable flux and reorganization in adolescence and early adulthood, followed by moderate stability in adulthood (the period for which Costa and colleagues have data). The transition into later life is quite stable for men, but marked by considerable reorganization of personality for women.

These two research programs show remarkable convergence of the traits found to be stable in men, and the Oakland studies provide a rare report of empirical data on personality development in women. Unfortunately, we have little guidance in what to expect of people as they develop past the age of 60. We also know that, in spite of objective stability in personality, people report believing that they have changed and grown (Bengtson, Reedy, & Gorden, 1985; Woodruff & Birren, 1972).

Another intriguing discussion in the study of personality development is the question of changes in gender role and stereotypic gender-based attitudes across the life span. David Gutmann

(1987), using projective testing in several cultures, has long argued that men and women cross over in later life, with women becoming more self-assertive and independent while men become more nurturing and caring. In a masterful review of the literature on self-concepts, Bengtson et al. (1985) conclude that findings are dependent on the method used to study the question: Objective personality measures tended to show more gender stereotypic patterns in earlier cohorts, whereas self-concept measures (e.g., the Bem Androgyny Scale) showed more androgyny in the older respondents. These authors also note that age-graded social roles and cohort effects are probable reasons for the reported differences and are very difficult to disentangle. There is, for example, some reason to believe that gender-based stereotyping in self-concept is strongest during the child-raising years, and that androgyny may be more common both before and after these years. In work with older adults, one should keep an open mind about the possibility of naturally occurring change in long-held behaviors and beliefs about gender-related issues. In fact, contrary to the popular image of older adults as holding fast to traditional gender roles and values, there may well be a tendency for men to become more interested in children and relationships and for women to become more interested in self-assertion, politics, and career.

Emotional changes over the adult life span are a topic of considerable importance for psychotherapists working with older adults. Gynther (1979), in a review of MMPI research with older adults, notes that older adults are lower on scales associated with anger, impulsivity, and confusion, and argues that we may become less impulsive with maturity. At the psychobiological level, Woodruff (1985) has concluded that older adults are more difficult to arouse, but also have more difficulty returning to a state of calm once aroused. This finding might suggest a different timeline for anxiety and anger in older adults than in younger ones. Schulz (1982) argued that the accumulation of experience leads to more complex and less extreme emotional experiences in later life. Each new experience reminds the older adults of previous experiences that may have a mix of negative and positive emotional connotations; whereas earlier in life it is possible to have simpler and more intense emotions, with little or no prior experience to moderate reactions, in response to new events (falling in love) or losses (a friend moving away).

Costa, Zonderman, McCrae, Cornoni-Huntley, Loke, and Barbano (1987), using a very large national sample, found evidence that average levels of life satisfaction stay stable with aging and across cohorts, but that earlier-born cohorts tend to express less positive and less negative affect. Labouvie-Vief, DeVoe, and Bulka (1989) propose a developmental model for the development of understanding the emotions and controlling the emotions, which moves from a very simple physical reaction and naming of feelings in early adolescence up to an integrated physical and emotional experience combined with an appreciation of situational determinants of the emotion and the reactions of others. This latter stage is reached in mid-life, according to their model. Malatesta and Izard (1984), reporting on the study of facial expression of emotions, discuss evidence that older people's expressions convey elements of several feelings at once. As a cautionary note to younger adults working with the elderly, they also report that younger people are much less accurate in identifying emotion in pictures of older faces. Taken as a whole, this body of work argues that emotionality in older adults will be more complex and more subtle than that of younger adults.

In general, clinical experience with older adults has led me to expect less expression of emotionality but a more complex mix of feelings more thoughtfully expressed. That is, older adults do, in fact, report feeling mixed reactions of happiness and sadness to the same event and can recall to memory many related past experiences, some that ended well and others with bad outcomes.

Life Satisfaction. Taking life satisfaction as a general measure of happiness and successful adjustment, life satisfaction research can provide some clues to ways to intervene with older adults to improve the mood of older clients. In general, the major determinants of life satisfaction for older adults are health, adequate income, and the presence of a confidant: a close relationship that includes self disclosure and emotional support (Botwinick, 1984). There is such a strong tendency to assume that problems of late life are due to isolation and loneliness, and that so activity and especially more social contact is an appropriate prescription for older clients, that several cautionary notes are in order. First, as described above (Costa et al., 1987), there actually is no evidence that older adults as a group are more unhappy than are younger adults as a group.

Second, preferences in activities, even at the level of simple leisure-time activities, are highly varied and related to personal style and needs (Tinsley, Teaff, Colbs, & Kaufman, 1985). Depending on the individual and his or her current needs, isolated activities (reading, gardening) may be more appropriate than group activity (bingo, dancing). One study in a large retirement village found that informal social contact was associated with positive mood, but participation in organized large-group activity actually led to lower life satisfaction (Longino & Kant, 1982). This specificity holds for contact with family members as well. Ward, Sherman, and LaGary (1984) found that frequent interaction with adult children was positive for older parents if the child was also a confidant. If the child was not considered a confidant, more contact led to lower levels of life satisfaction. The study of social interaction among the elderly has led to both an increasing appreciation of the costs of social contacts and the awareness that unpleasant social contacts increase depression (Rook, 1984).

All of this simply argues that the specific needs of the individual client and the specific circumstances of that client's interaction with family and friends must be carefully considered before encouraging increased activity, increased socialization, or even increased contact with families. While most therapists would take such a statement for granted with younger adults, when working with the elderly, many novices will switch to the simplistic, and inaccurate, assumption that all activity is good and all contact with family is positive.

Summary. In general, there is little reason to expect that psychotherapy will need much adaptation in working with the normally aging older person. Intelligence and memory change little in clinically relevant ways up to the age of 70 or so. Personality is relatively stable, with more continuity than change. Older people may, in fact, be more cognitively complex and more emotionally complex than younger adults. If these changes are combined with Neugarten's (1977) observation that interiority increases with age, older adults may be more suited for psychotherapy than younger adults, and certainly more interesting in their complexity.

Working with older adults may still be different and certainly may feel different. Among other things, cohort differences will be an issue whenever the therapist and client are from different cohorts. These differences may include different patterns of cognitive strengths and weaknesses, different educational levels and exposure to different models of education, different personality dispositions, different use of words, and certainly the whole complex of differing values and life experiences that comes from being of different times. This adaptation is not much different in kind or in degree from those required to work with clients of different social class, gender, or cultural background and is easy to overcome if understood correctly. Unfortunately, many professionals are sufficiently misinformed about aging to ascribe these kinds of differences to the aging process or to dementing illness and so consider these differences to be unchangeable and insurmountable.

The differences that I have previously described as being in the content of therapy (Knight, 1986) are, for many psychotherapists more difficult than I realized at that time. Being able to work effectively with persons who are chronically ill, disabled, dying, or grieving for others is specialized and demanding work. Many therapists find such work too emotionally difficult. A key element of the difference is changing from focusing on presumed potential in younger clients, with an optimistic spirit about their capacity for change, to having to work with problems that will not be changeable. In fact, the client's improvement often begins with the therapist's being able to say, "You will not recover previous eyesight," or "Your husband will never be back," and working through grief to the question of what comes next in life. This change is important but difficult for some therapists. In some cases, the difficulty may come from confronting such realities of life earlier than would be typical in the therapist's life course (cf. Knight, 1989); in other cases, it may come from personal issues in the individual therapist's life. In neither case does the problem lie in the client's age. These issues are more common in the latter third of life but are by no means specific to it.

Finally, therapy with the older adult can feel very difficult because it is very likely to call forth countertransference issues for the therapist. Working with older clients will evoke unresolved issues about parents and/or grandparents, and the way critical issues such as caring for an older relative were handled in one's family of origin, and will challenge the therapist's capacity to handle confrontation with death and with dependency due to chronic illness or disability. In my personal experience of doing psychotherapy and of teaching and consulting with others in the psychotherapy community, it seems to me that only family therapy so regularly confronts the therapist with issues from the past that are not yet resolved and with issues from the present and future not yet faced.

The Case Histories. The themes of similarities and differences in psychotherapy with the elderly are addressed case by case in the remainder of this book. After each case is presented, issues in building rapport with the client are discussed, followed by a description of what was done and any adaptation in usual therapeutic technique. The discussion continues by raising questions relating to the need for gerontological expertise and what the case may offer to the understanding of aging. Each chapter closes with a discussion of transference and countertransference issues as I now understand them.

Consistent with my hypothesis that therapy with older adults is distinctive mostly because of the greater prevalence of problems related to illness, grief, and dying, my initial selection of cases was guided by picking clients who illustrated one of these topic areas. Other clients were picked who had more general problems of anxiety, depression, sexual issues, and psychosis.

Case histories provide a greater sense of the reality of therapy than a general description of principles of psychotherapy with older adults possibly can. It is one thing to hear a general description of issues in working with older adults and another to hear the story of one person who embodies several problems at once.

Everyone who has read in gerontology has heard that we need a biopsychosocial model to cope with the multiple problems of the elderly. Hearing their personal life stories, however, drives home in a more immediate way that each client has a mix of medical, psychological, and social problems. In fact, a major lesson for me came from trying to organize the book. The cases do not, in fact, fit the description of the book's structure in the previous paragraph. Most stories in this volume illustrate several problems and several issues in therapy with older adults.

The case histories are presented as they occurred. It is my intention to try to give the facts first and then explain them. This approach should encourage and facilitate teaching about therapy by maximizing the reader's ability to second-guess. There are instances in which certain leads should have been followed up earlier. There are also times when important information emerges rather late in therapy. I have kept these accounts as veridical as possible to illustrate how denial, other forms of resistance, and the complexity of the lives of the elderly conspire to make the work interesting, challenging, and often surprising.

No matter how complete the initial history-taking and assessment are thought to be, more material will emerge later on. The sheer mass of life history material for the older client means that both therapist and client will have to make judgments about how much history needs to taken and what material is relevant to the current problem. As is true with all clients, some editing of the presented material will occur. Much of this editing will be emotionally motivated, intentionally or not. For example, it is not uncommon that a depressed older client who feels very lonely and unsupported will neglect to mention important friends and family contacts.

I have deliberately avoided describing assessments in detail. Assessment with the elderly is a specialized area and one that is worthy of another book. I have included the results of assessments and sometimes the rethinking of initial assessments that is an integral part of my approach to understanding clients. In my experience, initial assessments lead to therapy that often generates new information and reassessment.

Selection and Bias. Case histories are always selected and it is not always clear how or why. I have tried to avoid making myself look good. I have included cases that I do not consider successes. I have included cases that the client would not have considered a success. I have tried to avoid picking only interesting cases, which are interesting because they are atypical. I have tried to select a fairly broad and representative range of psychotherapy with older adults, as I have known it. I am aware that the cases misrepresent my work with older adults in one important way: Longer term cases are overrepresented. It is simply easier to remember, to contact, and to secure permission to write about clients I have known for a long time. There are short-term cases in this volume, but not as many as in my lifetime caseload of working with older adults. Some clients I would have very much liked to include declined the honor of being included.

Perhaps the most severe selection factor is that only one therapist is selected: myself. I will leave it to others to speculate on how that biases the selection of clients, the presentation of cases, and the conclusions drawn. I invite others to correct the problem by writing case histories of their own.

The cases are drawn from the scores of people I saw as a psychotherapist at the Senior Outreach program of Ventura County Mental Health. The program served people on a sliding scale fee basis, so ability to pay has not been a factor in cases. During the time that I worked there, fees were paid on an annual basis rather than on a session-by-session basis. Fees and length of therapy are thus independent of one another. We made extensive use of home visits and other outreach methods (cf. Knight, 1989). I have chosen to illustrate my argument that the site of therapy is irrelevant by not describing who was seen in which setting until the closing chapter. The outreach team included clinical social workers, clinical psychologists, mental health nurses, psychiatrists, and health educators. Ventura County has a sizable Hispanic minority group and small numbers of African-Americans and Asian-Americans. I have seen older people from these groups and invited some of them to be written about; they have declined.

The fact that the program is in Southern California accounts for the scarcity of sessions with several family members present. Most of the clients described here were living a considerable distance from family. The experience of working with large numbers of older adults who have moved such distances to live in Southern California, and their disappointment with the results of that move, undoubtedly account for some of the opinions expressed about the wisdom of relocating. Experiences in other places may be quite different.

With this general background, the presentation of case histories begins. The reader is invited and encouraged to second-guess, re-conceptualize, and speculate about the clients and the therapist. It is my hope that the book will serve as a window into the usually closed consultation room of the psychotherapist, in this instance one who is working with older clients.

CHAPTER ONE

Harold, an Artist and Teacher:
Enjoyment and Depression

Harold was in his early 80s and relatively healthy. He had chronic heart problems for which he took medication. He had moved to California from the East Coast about 2 years prior to coming in for therapy. He was referred by his physician following a suicide attempt in which he had taken a large quantity of his heart medication and some antidepressants. The dose was large enough to have been fatal or nearly so. However, he had rather quickly "lost his nerve" and told his wife what he had done and she drove him to the emergency room of a local hospital. His wife was 5 years older, and they had been arguing earlier that evening. After this suicide attempt, the physician had reevaluated his medical condition and the risk of using medication for suicide, discontinued the medication, and referred him for psychotherapy.

He initially reported his major problem as simply being bored. He had been very active as an artist and in teaching art when he lived in a small university town in the East. After moving to Ventura County, he had found it sufficiently large to make finding new friends difficult, but not large enough to have the kind of artistic community he had hoped to find. He had attempted to connect with local schools of art but had failed to do so. He attributed the failure to either having differing interests, differing teaching philosophies, or to what he perceived as failing ability on his part. He also felt that his wife restricted him in that they had different interests, her health was failing, and she was jealous of any separate activities. Since many of his complaints and restrictions involved his wife, couples sessions were suggested. He felt she would refuse, and in fact she did so politely a few months later, when we had arranged a visit for memory assessment and to present her view of him.

He also worried about memory impairment and declining abilities. Memory assessment revealed no testable impairment. While at his level of education and intelligence this result is not conclusive, he was unable to identify any precise areas in which memory or other cognitive abilities were sufficiently worse to require him to change activities. He had, in fact, purchased a computer and was learning word-processing and database software. Over the course of several weeks of therapy, it seemed that this concern about his ability was a continuation of a lifelong self-criticism. His low self-esteem had been counteracted in mid-life by the admiration of students, colleagues, and admirers, none of whom had followed him westward.

He also constantly portrayed his wife as physically frail but more alert that he. When she came in a few months later, it developed that she was mildly to moderately memory-impaired and more worried about his physical health than his cognitive abilities. She related that he sometimes pushed himself too hard on his daily walks and had passed out several blocks from home on occasion.

Regardless of cause, he continued to refuse to seek opportunities to teach and mostly refused to practice his art. He needed models and was too shy and too fearful of failure to seek out any. He fantasized about conversational relationships with young women, but portrayed his wife as too jealous to permit this. He denied sexual interest in younger women, although he talked of wanting to take classes with nude live models. He found reasons not to do this as well. He had one male friend, also an artist, whom he enjoyed but whom he felt was too busy to see him often. He had one son who lived out of state whom he portrayed as emotionally distant, although the son did make time for a month-long trip to Mexico with his father.

From the viewpoint of a therapy aimed at increased enjoyment, Harold presented an interesting challenge in that, while he and the therapist could easily identify numerous activities that he had found highly enjoyable in the past, he could equally easily find reasons not to do any of them. After considerable discussion over several weeks, with many failed "homework assignments," he did make a connection with a small local church with an intellectually oriented congregation. He did some artwork for the church and also struck up a sustaining relationship with the young, female minister. His depression was considerably alleviated after this. He was never again suicidal, stating that his first experience at attempting to kill himself convinced him that it was not as good an idea as he had imagined.

He also eventually came to see his reluctance to resume art or teaching as a decision rather than as due to failed ability. He attributed his self-criticism to a very critical father who had been a blue-collar worker and generally scornful of his son's artistic ambition. This negative influence had been counterbalanced by forceful teachers who had compelled him to continue working and show his work.

He also came to reinterpret his wife's jealousy and other barriers that she put in his way as his way of excusing his own shyness. He acknowledged that he could in fact pursue his interests if he wanted to. We terminated therapy after having been at a plateau for a couple of months in which he was still dissatisfied with his life, unwilling to make any changes in it, but no longer clinically depressed.

I saw him a few times more than a year later, at which point he had acknowledged that his wife, now severely demented, had been cognitively impaired for a number of years and that he had been denying this.

DISCUSSION

Harold provides an interesting challenge for discussion in that, in many ways, he would seem one of the best suited for therapy of the clients presented in this volume, but he made rather limited use of therapy and left improved but not entirely successful.

Rapport Building. Harold came to therapy willingly and affably, but with an undercurrent of reserve. He initially perceived the visits as a combination of punishment for his rash action in taking the overdose and as a way of reassuring his wife and his doctor that he would not do it again. He needed no education about the nature of therapy and very little about the nature of depression. He was highly verbal and willing to talk about his problems in adjusting to California.

At the same time, his acceptance of therapy and of me was rather shallow. He was truly lonely and dissatisfied with his life; however, he expressed very little emotional pain or intense distress. His life was empty but not painful.

Techniques in Therapy. After assessment verified no significant cognitive or physical impairment and a lack of current suicidal intention, Harold seemed a prime candidate for a cognitive-behavioral intervention, focused on redefining himself as a competent person and on increasing the number of pleasant events in his life, following Peter Lewinsohn's analysis of depression as maintained by the reduced number of pleasant events (positive reinforcers) in the depressed person's life (cf. Lewinsohn & McPhillamy, 1974; Lewinsohn, Munoz, Youngren, & Zeiss, 1978).

Identifying his personal array of pleasant events was quite easy: He enjoyed art, intellectual conversation, talking to young women, teaching, writing, and socializing. All of these had clearly been rewarding in the past, and his eyes would light up and he would become more animated as he talked about them in the present. He was, however, very resistant to follow through on his assignments to resume any of these activities. My response to this resistance was to lower the task demands: Rather than trying to take on a paid assignment or even a self-assigned series of artistic studies, the homework would be to sit in front of the easel for a half hour sometime this week. I also kept reassigning the same pleasures, or asked him to select a new one that would be easier, while maintaining a nonjudgmental stance about his noncompletions: "That's what it's like to be depressed; change is really difficult, it will take a while." As noted, after several weeks of this, he increased his time doing art and became involved in a local church group.

In terms of challenging his perception of himself as disabled, the technique worked but the result was mixed. As we repeatedly discussed various situations in which he saw himself as incompetent or disabled, it was always possible to rephrase his concerns in less negative and depression-evoking terms. This level of reinterpretation can be seen as consistent with any of the cognitive therapies (Beck, Ellis's rational-emotive, Kelly's [1955] personal constructs). Success in carrying out pleasant events can be seen as increasing self-efficacy (Bandura, 1982). In one sense this worked; Harold quit seeing himself as developing dementia or as "too old" to pursue his interests. What emerged instead was a portrayal of himself as passive and self-doubting throughout his life, beginning with the excessive criticism of his father. In retrospect, he saw himself as forced into the art world by an aggressive and dominant mentor and then constantly admired by colleagues, his students, and his wife. Retirement and a somewhat shallowly considered move to California deprived him of these external reinforcers and external corrections of his negative internal self-perception and left him with his lifelong sense of inferiority. While he could intellectually appreciate that his life disproved this negative perception of himself, this cognitive restructuring had no apparent emotional impact.

I have said little about the change in his suicidality because I believe that this change occurred before therapy. Like most of the old-old, Harold had no fear of death and in many ways looked forward to it. Like all too many who are living the postretirement life-style, he had had a rather romanticized notion of suicide as an alternative to the boredom of his life. His attempt itself changed this conception: As he felt himself weaken, he realized that he wanted to live and that suicide was not going to be as pleasant as he had imagined. Fortunately for him, he had chosen a method that allowed time to reconsider and he also had someone closeby to take him for treatment.

His marriage had also improved in that he had come to accept that most of his unhappiness was under his control, rather than to be blamed on his wife, and so their daily arguments and complaining reduced considerably. Unfortunately, he also learned, from assessment process and from her continued decline, that his wife was dementing and becoming more dependent on him. He rose to this challenge rather well, and it seemed easier to accept his wife as cognitively impaired rather than seeing her as withholding her former supportiveness, being jealous, and being intentionally critical of him.

Gerontological Issues. Age-specific expertise comes into play in this case primarily in the assessment and in the ability to make appropriate referrals for his increasing involvement in the community. Harold came in articulating concerns about failing ability and failing memory. The ability to assess these complaints was essential to starting therapy and to restructuring Harold's own perception of these changes. This assessment included a standard mental status examination (Folstein, Folstein, & McHugh, 1975), subtests from the Wechsler Memory Scale, and thorough examination of the situations that prompted his complaints. I suspect that someone lacking in gerontological expertise would have either accepted his complaints at face value or dismissed them without investigation, and that neither approach would have satisfied Harold.

Knowledge of the local aging network of services and activities led to very limited discussion of those possibilities with Harold. I never, for example, suggested either senior recreation centers or any of our local senior volunteer programs as an alternative, since all were oriented to a lower level of education and artistic talent. The two programs that did have intellectual appeal he had already checked out and found lacking. In fact, Harold's increased activity was all in age-integrated settings and mostly with younger people.

Harold also illustrates a common problem in serving older adults. It is easy to say that someone who is isolated and alone needs to socialize, but overcoming the internal barriers to such socialization may require considerable individual work. The isolation of the elderly is often conceptualized as due to lack of opportunity to interact. Harold illustrates Rook's (1984) contention that there are often personological reasons for such isolation that must be taken into consideration. In Harold's case, lifelong passivity, inferiority, and introversion made socializing difficult. His own decision to leave familiar surroundings, and his highly selective stance toward social contacts, limited his opportunity.

Relationship Issues. Harold evidenced a generally positive feeling for me and over time challenged the limits of the therapeutic relationship with various indications that he would rather that I be a friend. Although in part sincere, I believe that this was also a positively toned form of resistance on his part: Asking that I be his friend was also a way of asking that I back off in encouraging him to change.

Similarly, for me Harold was a positive figure who evoked images of conversations with my father and with professors I had liked. To my knowledge, this had little impact on the course of therapy, except for needing to monitor more carefully his attempts to distract me into pleasant but nontherapeutic conversation than was true with many other clients. I found his invitations to friendship attractive, but never felt this was in any way an option since his therapy was never, and in my opinion is still not, completed.

Summary. In conclusion, Harold represents an example of modest success of cognitive behavioral approaches with a more than 80-year-old man. He was improved at the end of therapy, but had clearly neither reached his initial goals nor redefined those goals. It appears that this limited success is due to his decision to stop working on change, rather than on any limitation of the technique.

CHAPTER TWO

Helen:
Life Review and Depression

When she started therapy, Helen was not quite 60, unemployed, and living with her parents. Her father had been taking care of her mother, who was reported to have been moderately to severely demented for a number of years. Her mother also had arthritis and osteoporosis. Her father was described as a small man with severe curvature of the spine and a bad heart condition. He was also subject to periodic bouts of severe depression.

She described herself as assisting her father in his care of her mother. However, as she talked in more detail, it emerged that she could more accurately be described as taking care of both of them. Her parents argued and yelled at one another quite often, a continuation of a lifelong pattern but one that she had not been regularly exposed to since her teenage years. Her mother at this time was suspicious of both of them, accusing them of taking her money and plotting to kill her. Helen also found her father's depression overwhelming and contagious, especially since she had a prior history of treatment for depression herself.

Her situation was also complicated by relative isolation from friends, in that she had lived much of her adult life in Los Angeles and most of her friends were there rather than in Ventura County. After moving, she had worked for a while for a juvenile corrections center, but her job had been eliminated in cutbacks after the tax revolt initiative in California. Her father had encouraged her simply to live with them and help. While financially convenient, it left her not only dependent on her parents but also without outside structured activity or support for her self-esteem.

When she first came in, she was severely depressed at times and moderately depressed chronically. She felt fatigued and described her situation as being hopeless and felt helpless to change it. She worried about her own mental abilities and feared that she would follow her mother into dementia. The only reported cognitive changes were better understood as problems in concentration and decision making, which are common to depression. For example, she often was unable to finish a book or a magazine article and would become quite confused trying to decide what she could do with her life now. She expressed considerable guilt about not doing more for her parents, not working, and having negative feelings toward her parents, who were both quite ill and disabled.

She thought often about death, usually in an abstract way, but more recently had incidents in which she started planning to kill herself. Further exploration of this revealed relatively indefinite plans: She had no target date and thought that the means would either be an ancient gun that she thought her father owned or some pills, which she did not have and did not know what kind she would use. She had had suicidal impulses in the past in conjunction with other depressions and could recall having been taken to the emergency room and admitted to a psychiatric hospital on one occasion, but felt that she had not, in fact, been close to dying from the attempt. She had trouble sleeping at night and then would often be lethargic and sit in one chair most of the day. She tended to overeat when depressed and had been gaining weight.

On the third visit, we discussed referring her to the team psychiatrist for antidepressant medication. Her objections centered on a prior bad experience with lithium. Careful questioning failed to reveal any clear history of manic episodes, although this interview did reveal an admission to a psychiatric day-treatment program several years earlier. She consented to see the psychiatrist after we reassured her that we would not duplicate her experience with lithium toxicity, which had resulted in acute confusion and a residual hand tremor that lasted several months after the lithium was discontinued. She was started on relatively low doses of an antidepressant and carefully monitored for possible manic changes. The psychiatrist felt that some of her history was suggestive of hypomanic episodes, although no clear manic episode was described by Helen or noted in the records we received from her previous psychiatrist.

Our early sessions focused primarily on allowing Helen to talk about her current situation and her feelings about it. She found considerable initial relief (over a period of 2 to 3 months) in simply being able to talk to someone other than her parents about the situation she found herself in. I also encouraged her to express her feelings of depression, her sense of being trapped, and her anxiety about her future. She would also express her sense of guilt about having such feelings, to which my response was assurance that it was natural to have complex and negative feelings, given the situation.

We also explored alternative solutions to the family situation. She saw her mother's condition as hopeless and overwhelming to her father. A home visit by other members of the outreach team confirmed this picture as well as her description of her father as intensely depressed. Her father refused therapy and also refused to see his doctor in response to Helen's concerns about his physical health. He was also adamant about keeping his wife at home until the end.

We explored ways she could find support outside the home, and this did lead to renewed contacts with old friends in the Los Angeles area. As a way to bolster self-esteem, as well as learn more about her, we spent time talking about her job in juvenile corrections. She had taken considerable pride in her work, both in her ability to establish rapport with difficult kids and in her ability to intuit when they were lying or planning something, and so she was able to discipline them effectively and win their respect.

While these early sessions and the medication seemed to result in some improvement of her feelings of distress and alleviation of her depression, she remained significantly depressed and would periodically hit periods of especially depressed mood. She would report these primarily in terms of comments from other people, times of feeling very tired, or the return of thinking about death constantly even though her circumstances had changed very little. Her depression would often be a surprise to her in that she had very little sense of becoming more depressed or would scarcely noticed it until someone commented on her appearance or she noticed her own inactivity. She was frightened by this inability to see the depression coming and wondered if she might become impulsively suicidal in the same way. It also posed a problem for her use of medication, which she needed to adjust by her mood, since any given dosage seemed sometimes to produce a mild hypomania and at other times be insufficient to prevent depression. This problem prompted the use of some daily monitoring of her moods so that she could learn to understand and predict her feelings.

She experienced some improvement in her ability to identify her feelings and track her depression over time. One night she heard her father call her name. She went to the living room to find him complaining of some pain in his chest. She called the ambulance, but he died before it arrived.

After the immediate sense of shock and disbelief, along with the busywork of funeral preparations and visits from friends and family, her primary reactions were anger and guilt. We reviewed a number of times her efforts to get him to seek help from their physician and from our outreach team. We also reviewed a number of times the death night itself, as she sought out something that she could have done differently that would have kept her father alive. She began to experience her anger that he had refused help and that he had left her alone with her mother.

In talking about her father and her relationship with him, it came out that as a child she had felt responsible for protecting her mother from him. Her father had been distant from her but often hostile toward the mother, including both verbal abuse and physical fights. As a young adult, Helen had once hit him with a frying pan to keep him from attacking her mother. After that, she had distanced herself from both of them. They had later divorced, married other people, divorced those people, and remarried. She described her shock and disbelief when they called to tell her they were back together again. She had remained distant from them until her mother's illness aroused her sense of responsibility to care for them. She felt that age and disability had mellowed her father and that they had forgiven one another for past events, although he had remained a distant, cold man.

Moving into the primary caregiver role with only one parent to focus on, she directed her concerns toward learning about Alzheimer's disease and ways to better care for her mother. She became active for a while in the ADRDA chapter and learned a lot that was helpful in caregiving tasks and in taking care of legal and financial management issues. With her father's death, all property and money had passed to her mother, who had no idea what she owned and, in fact, had to be reminded constantly that her husband had died. Even though it was a difficult time, Helen's mood seemed to become stable at a mildly depressed level. At one point, months after his death, she was able to verbalize that there was some sense of relief in having only one parent to care for.

There were still times of intense depression, guilt, and thoughts of death. During one of these she called me at the office to report that she was sitting on the sofa and staring at her father's gun, which she had found and which was now on top of the television: "I'm not sure what I'm going to do." After some discussion to establish that she felt able to follow these directions, we agreed that she would put the gun in a bag, put it in the trunk of her car, and come to my office. She asked a neighbor to watch her mother for an hour or so. She came in and gave me the gun. We talked about her mood and her sense of feeling suicidal, which passed fairly quickly. She felt safe as long as the gun was out of the house. With a contract that she would call me if the impulses returned before our next scheduled visit, she returned home.

For the next several weeks, sessions focused on occasional suicidal impulses and on a more persistent desire to die. She felt trapped by needing to care for her mother and saw no escape from the situation. She felt an obligation to both parents to keep her mother at home. She also felt that placing her in a nursing home was financially impossible. She was unemployed and too young by a couple of years for Social Security, so the only source of income and housing was her mother's pension and the family home, presently in both names. She was also convinced that she was going to become demented like her mother and that her mother was likely to outlive her. Death appeared to be the only escape.

In response to a comment that she thought her mother would be very pleased to have her in this situation and under such tight control, if only she could comprehend that it had happened, we began to explore the history of her relationship with her mother. It emerged that she had not felt close to her mother, even though she had been in the role of her mother's protector since childhood. Her mother was described as domineering, intrusive, jealous, and demanding. Her mother's behavior was seen by neighbors as eccentric. In fact, she was perceived as "the peculiar one" in a family of origin that was eccentric and proud of it. Helen had withdrawn as much as possible, but even when quiet and reading, she would be accused of thinking up things to do to her mother. Punishment was unpredictable and swift.

An early attempt to escape by marrying a young man in the military was thwarted when the mother went after her and brought her home from the military base. Her mother interfered in her raising her son. It was only after she divorced and left the area that she achieved some independence. Finding herself once again as her mother's caregiver gave Helen the feeling that her mother had won a lifelong struggle between them.

Reevaluating this chain of events, in terms of Helen's motives rather than her mother's, led to perceiving this as an effort on her part to come to terms with her difficult parents before they died. She felt modestly successful in this effort with her father, but came to realize that it was too late with her mother, who was now almost nonverbal and had very little memory of her own history. Helen was able to grieve for this lost opportunity and to achieve some closure by some "what if" conversations in therapy sessions, with her imagining what it would have been like to talk things through with her mother. Her conclusion was that her mother would never have changed. This conclusion did enable her to give up the attempt to resolve this part of her life.

With this work done in therapy, she began to explore ways of getting her mother into a nursing home. She found a solution that got her mother into an acceptable home on MediCal and allowed her to keep the family home, but it did involve a waiting period of more than a year. During this time we continued to work on improved monitoring and control of her depressions and explored what she would do when her mother was out of the home. The monitoring of her moods led to two cues: an excessive eating of sweets, which also potentiated her depressions since she was hypoglycemic, and a concerned look on her dog's face. With these cues in mind, she was able to identify the onset of severe depressions a few days in advance and ameliorate it by not binging on sweets and by taking increased doses of her antidepressant medication.

With her mother in the nursing home, she gradually began to reestablish a sense of who she was after 4 years of being a caregiver to her parents. We reviewed her work history in social services, rediscovering her sense of pride in her accomplishments. She found some volunteer work in social services and worked part-time for a while in a shelter for homeless women. She also became involved again in feminist political action groups and joined a progressive church group that had a kind of nonreligious emphasis on self-improvement. She decided to set a goal of moving to a small desert community she had enjoyed visiting as a child, and was able to do so several years later. Until that time, she maintained contact with infrequent office visits and group therapy, increasing the visits during times of crisis in the lives of her sons.

DISCUSSION

Rapport Building.   Helen was unusual in that she was very ready for therapy. She had prior experience with psychotherapy and had some college-level course work in psychology. She was an avid reader in general and had read several works by well-known therapists as well as novels about the therapeutic experience. In her specific case, there was no problem in initial rapport building or orientation to therapy. If anything, the problem was that she was too knowledgeable and able to play the ideal client without becoming engaged in the work of therapy.

Techniques in Therapy.   Helen's therapy divides into three distinct phases: the initial work prior to the death of her father, with a focus on depression and the stresses of caring for both parents; the grief work and life review following her father's death; and finally the focus on prediction of mood swings after the life review was completed.

The first phase departs from other approaches to depression described in this book in that it relied largely on ventilation of emotion and a problem-solving approach, rather than an attempt to increase pleasure or restructure her thinking. Both the context of family caregiving and the obvious emotional tension with which she presented called for a stress reduction model as an initial therapeutic strategy. Borrowing from crisis intervention models of psychotherapy (Ewing, 1978), this approach recognizes the need to allow for expression of emotion and address immediate problems in a collaborative problem-solving mode. The crisis intervention approach is often helpful in working with older adults in severe stress, even though the "crisis" is quite often a chronic stressor, like caregiving, rather than an acute, discrete stress event such as might be seen with younger adults (cf. Pearlin et al., 1990).

In this sense, stress reduction calls for both allowing and encouraging expression of emotions in an active listening mode. In Helen's instance, this often involved a need to encourage her to focus on emotions, rather than day-to-day problems and arguments, and to assist her in identifying some emotions. After a few sessions of this work, emotional release was mixed with not only understanding how the stressful situation had evolved and what the components of the stress were, but also considering alternatives to reduce her level of stress.

In her particular instance, much of the stress came from her high expectations for herself as a caregiver for her parents. These expectations were rather clearly held by her parents as well. Many of their expectations were of the double-bind type; that is, they would state an expectation and then frustrate her attempts to satisfy it. For example, she was expected to keep her father healthy, and yet he consistently refused to see doctors whom she had found for him. Rediscovering this pattern and letting herself off the hook was an important part of her feeling less distressed by caring for her parents.

An obvious question, of course, is why she stayed in this situation. The answer was in part financial. She had left her job to take care of them and was now unmotivated to seek work again. She was in her late 50s and thought that caring for her parents would last until she qualified for Social Security at age 62. From a stress management viewpoint, the important element of this is that she had made and was continuing to make a choice to take care of her parents. The alternative was seen as even more stressful, because she had last worked as a probation officer.

She was experiencing partial relief from stress when her father died. This event naturally changed the course of therapy into grief work for her father. She felt considerable guilt, and we examined the night of his death a number of times. She fairly quickly concluded that there was nothing else she could have done, but did worry for some time that she should have heard him sooner, should not have been sleeping, and so on. She also wrestled with feeling guilt for not somehow making him go to a doctor (cf. Worden, 1982). Again, it was realistically difficult to see how she could have done any more than she had in this regard. In addition, it seemed predictable that even if he had seen a doctor, he would not have followed any treatment plan for more than a few days. As it often does, the grief work led to life review. Much of the information already reported about her relationship with her father, and his with her mother, came up in therapy as she struggled to find an appropriate way to feel about the death of her father, to whom she had never felt very close and with whom she had often fought.

Her father's death also posed new tasks for Helen. He had been cognitively intact and in charge of the finances. Her mother was quite demented, so Helen had to take over paying bills, keeping track of savings, and planning for their future. She also came to realize how much her father had been doing for her mother: work that she now had to take over by herself. These realizations not only were examples of the adjustment to new roles, which is part of grief work, but also served to initiate a period of grieving for her mother. By this time, the older woman was almost nonverbal and often thought Helen was either her sister or an unrelated nice woman who did things for her. As she reviewed her relationship with her father, she also slowly came to recognize that her mother was gone, too, even though still living. This realization, once complete, led to less stress and to a decision to place her mother in 24-hour care as soon as possible. Due to their financial situation and to MediCal regulations, this proved to involve a 2-year waiting period. She never escaped the feeling that her mother had won an ironic victory over her: that she was trapped in caring for her mother who would have enjoyed the situation immensely, had she still been cognitively intact.

As her stress lessened and her grief resolved, Helen's mood swings became more apparent. Since we never saw nor had report of a full manic episode, we had diagnosed her as cyclothymic. She would have brief periods of elation and high levels of activity, long periods of normal mood, and short periods of intense depression with thoughts of death and a pervasive sense of despair. These patterns tended to follow an annual cycle, with longer periods of depression in October and April. She initially was unable to track these mood swings, nor was she able to notice them coming on: She would simply find herself in the depths.

Based on my conviction that they must have a noticeable pattern, and that knowing the pattern would increase her control, we initiated self-monitoring of mood levels and kept a diary of daily mood ratings and activities (cf. Goldfried & Davison, 1976). This record eventually led to her discovery that she binged on chocolates before becoming intensely depressed. After discovering this, she also recalled that she had been diagnosed as hypoglycemic several years earlier. With yet more record keeping, she was able to notice other cues (e.g., a look of concern on her dog's face; declining neatness in the house) and even more slowly actually began to notice smaller changes in her moods. She was then able to use these other cues to adjust her medication and take other steps to prevent depression. Older adults with severe mood swings often have this inability to recognize their emotional states, and self-monitoring helps them to develop this skill and gain better control over mood swings.

Gerontological Issues. Since Helen turned 60 while I was seeing her in therapy, she was not, strictly speaking, a gerontology case. In fact, I considered her to be included as a child caring for elderly parents. In that context, some knowledge of the aging process and of the caregiving literature was helpful in working with her. (For more reading on caregiving issues, see Light & Lebowitz, 1990; Mace & Rabins, 1982; Zarit, Orr, & Zarit, 1985.) In the earlier part of that work, educating Helen to focus on the diseases that her parents had and what could and could not be done to help them, as opposed to focusing on their age and accepting everything that happened as normal for this phase of life, helped to improve both her care of them and her sense of well-being. She had been assuming that her parents were models of her own future aging; later she was more realistically concerned about her risk of developing similar illnesses. This concern for her own health led to increased doctor visits for herself, greater concern for nutrition, and some attempts to reduce and control her weight.

The need to grieve for her father after his death and for her mother prior to her physical death is a frequent and important part of working with the elderly. As Helen's therapy illustrates, grief work often involves life review and the review of life with the departed. She was impelled to review her life, her life with each parent, what she knew of each parent's life, and their life together as a couple. This process is part of reconstructing a life without the deceased loved one in it (Rando, 1984; Worden, 1982). This mass of material brought considerable clarity to why she was doing what she was doing and to why she found it so difficult.

She had a lifelong struggle with her parents as individuals and as a couple, and they were, in fact, difficult people with a mostly dysfunctional relationship. At 60, Helen began to consider and accept the idea that her parents were limited people with little to offer her, as opposed to powerful people who had withheld much from her. Her review of life with her mother led her to see their relationship as a long battle, one that would not be resolved now that her mother was dementing, and probably would not have been resolved in any case. The ability to work within a life span perspective and analyze patterns in relationships that span decades is an important aspect of working with older adults that is missing in work with the young.

On the other hand, individual cases like Helen's suggest a richness of ambivalence and complexity in the experience of being a caregiver for older parents that is missing from virtually all accounts of caregiving in both the gerontological and popular literatures, both of which tend to portray family caregiving as the only problem occurring in otherwise loving and well-balanced families.

In many ways, the real impact of gerontological expertise in working with Helen was in not seeing her as "an aging case." While she was concerned about growing old and becoming limited in various ways, I saw her as quite young, with a long life ahead of her. This viewpoint changed the way that she perceived herself, and the way she made different decisions about her life. Specifically, she decided to return to work for a while, did some long-term financial planning, and based her care for her mother on the assumption that they both had indefinite but quite likely fairly long lives ahead of them and that hers would be longer than her mother's. (At the beginning of therapy, some of her inaction was based on the passive hope that she [Helen] would die soon.)

In another sense, neither the response to her suicidal thoughts nor the treatment plan for handling her mood swings was based on a perception of her as "geriatric." Instead, we followed regular mental health treatment plans and worked with her as we would an adult of any age. Our gerontological expertise shows only in that we had no hesitation in pursuing such plans based on her age.

Relationship Issues. Helen's relationship to me was generally positive and largely uncomplicated by transferential issues. Through most of the therapy, I believe that her past experience with psychotherapists and with psychiatrists kept me in a rather realistic and appropriate role in her life. Toward the end, I think there may have been some tendency to identify me with her older son, who was about my age and on whom she relied for advice and with whom she discussed her life quite openly. It does not appear to me that this transference distorted the therapy, although it may have prolonged it.

On my side, there was considerable positive feeling for Helen. She was one of the brighter and funnier clients that I had. We shared a similar sense of humor and view of the world. Especially after her suicidal crisis, I came to feel somewhat responsible for her. Although it was a threat, it seemed to me then (and now) that it was one of the few really serious threats I have heard, and I think of Helen as one of the very few people whom I saved from suicide. This feeling deepened the sense of attachment I felt to her and gave me a possibly unrealistic sense of responsibility for her.

I have a suspicion that these factors caused me to prolong the therapy with her more than I might have done with someone else. My rationale (or rationalization) was and is that she was under considerable chronic stress, first while caring for her mother and later in relating to family problems with her sons, and that there was no point at which termination seemed appropriate. The issues with her sons emerged only after her mother was placed. Prior to that, one was largely absent from her life and the other was supportive in practical ways when he was able to visit. After her mother was placed, they were in more frequent contact and she became concerned with their problems. This material occurred later in therapy than the sessions presented in this chapter.

We did discuss termination on several occasions but always agreed that there were still problems that needed work. Therapy became less frequent and later on shifted to a group context. We did not end therapy, however, until she moved out of the area and I took a different job. While I can still defend each individual decision to continue the therapy, it seems to me now that the total length can be best explained as due to the mutual positive bonding between us, rather than to the specific problems that served as a rationale for continuing.

Helen's therapy raised a different kind of ethical dilemma for me as well. The program in which I saw her, like most community-based programs for older adults, had a commitment to maintaining the elderly in the community. It was initially my belief that providing psychotherapy for caregivers would tend to achieve this objective by reducing the stress of the caregivers and enabling them to care for the patients longer in the community. It became clear to me fairly early in my work with Helen that reducing her stress, and especially the guilt that caused much of her stress, was likely to lead to her placing her mother in a nursing home earlier, rather than prolonging at-home care. It also was clear to me that this would be a positive outcome for Helen. It was equally clear that if her mother had been my client, I would likely have been advocating for continued home care. Certainly, the early placement of her mother would be a tally mark on the failure side for the programmatic goal of maintaining older people in the community, reducing public sector costs, and so on. I have already reported what I did; here I wish to call attention to the unresolved ethical dilemma and to the fact that the institutional care versus community care decision is seldom much more simple than this and usually does involve competing interests among the family members involved.

Summary. Helen's therapy lasted several years and embraced numerous themes and issues in work with older adults: caregiving, grieving, chronic illness, deciding to place a parent in a nursing home, and life review. The interconnectedness of these problems in one person's life is difficult to appreciate without such specific real-life examples. One of the dissatisfactions I felt with my previous book on psychotherapy is that devoting a chapter to each of these problems leaves one with the feeling that they are conceptually separate and happen to different people.

The adult life span is also continuous. Helen's problems were not only "aging problems," but were also occurring within the context of not only a decades-long struggle with severely oscillating moods but also a lifelong history of struggling with a very dysfunctional family of origin. The dialectical tension of blending aging expertise and psychotherapy is best captured in such individual cases that illustrate working with late-life issues while continuing to be alert to psychological disorders and familial dysfunction.

CHAPTER THREE

John:
Enjoyment and Depression With Disabilities

I met John through his wife, whom I had seen for several sessions
for stress related to caring for him. After a couple of months of her
own therapy, she had suggested that I see John to determine if I
thought he might be depressed. This request surprised me because she had described him as extremely impaired physically
and cognitively. After some discussion, we established that she
now saw him as physically impaired but still verbal enough and
bright enough to communicate.

When I first saw him, the immediate impression was of extreme
frailty. He was in his late 60s but was unusually frail for his age,
having suffered a series of debilitating strokes. He was small, had
lost considerable weight, had extremely poor vision, was very
hard of hearing, and spoke very softly. Verbal communication
was difficult, but possible if I sat very close to him on the side of
his good ear. I also had to lean forward to catch his voice, which
was often at the level of a faint whisper. Occasionally, key words
would prove difficult to get across, and one of us would have to
write a word or a short phrase to the other.

Mental status examination showed no more than a slight memory impairment at this stage. The diagnostic interview confirmed
good memory for his life history as well as an accurate sense of
what his wife had gone through in caring for him. He had good
insight into their relationship and showed flashes of humor about
his condition and their marriage, which had often been stormy.
He also, not surprisingly, showed considerable depression. He
was sad, felt both hopeless and helpless, regarded his life as essentially over, and had suicidal thoughts but felt helpless to act on
them. His appetite and sleep were poor. He felt angry about his

helplessness and dependence on his wife and had no way (in his view) to express those feelings since he felt that she was nearly overwhelmed and close to leaving him as it was.

John had been an alcoholic and a gambler and had given up both with the help of Alcoholics Anonymous and Gamblers Anonymous. He had been very active in both self-help groups, with a wide network of friends and supporters, but these had faded away during his lengthy disability. Since he had moved out of Los Angeles to Ventura, he had virtually no contact with these friends. He rarely left the house, since he walked very slowly with canes and needed his wife's assistance. He described himself as unable to drive, read, write, or watch television. He retained a social and engaging demeanor. He was willing to give therapy a try, partly because he felt that his wife was feeling better since coming in and partly because he had nothing else to do.

The early phase of therapy consisted of learning to communicate with one another and with my encouraging him to describe his view of his condition and his feelings about it. Neither of these tasks came easily to him. He was acutely aware of the impact of his illness on his wife and was inclined to phrase everything in terms of its impact on her. Thus his inability to walk was a hardship for his wife. His wife found it difficult to watch him eat and became impatient because he was slow. His wife was frustrated with his inability to communicate. His wife felt he should try to do more and "fight back" against his disabilities.

All of these observations were true, and in some ways his concern for his wife and her responses to him were an important part of maintaining their relationship. Nonetheless, these first sessions focused on getting him to talk about the impact of these problems on himself. Accomplishing this required sentence-by-sentence interruption and editing. While this is often true, it felt different to be interrupting and challenging the speech of a client for whom speaking was tiring and very difficult physically. Nonetheless, John changed what he talked about and almost immediately began to feel and express considerable anger and depression about his disabilities.

He obtained some relief simply from emotional expression; however, this relief seemed to highlight the very boring nature of his days. From the description above, it can be seen that his days were boring and that ways to change them were far from obvious. In one sense, the very extremity of his circumstances suggested a sense of hope, since almost any change was likely to bring significant improvement.

The next stage, lasting several sessions, involved learning about what he had enjoyed doing prior to his illness. Much of this review led to more anger and depression, gradually resolving into acceptance of his new circumstances. Clearly he would not drive again, would not play a leadership role in the self-help movement again, would not even be able to attend meetings regularly again. For a man whose whole life had revolved around social activities, these limitations were devastating and required considerable adjustment. His wife was unable to listen to him grieve for these losses or express anger over losing this part of his life. She was grieving the loss of the husband who was extremely capable and social and she also construed such talk as self-defeating for him. In his few contacts with former friends and associates, they too regarded any such expression as pessimism or negative thinking on his part. In John's world, therapy provided the only outlet for talking honestly about the rather natural depression and anger over having lost most of his abilities without hope of recovering to pre-stroke levels.

A few activities emerged that it seemed could be resumed at some level. He had very much enjoyed listening to music and had given it up because he found regular radio very difficult to hear, especially if there were any distracting background noise. Buying a radio/tape player with earphones solved this problem and introduced some pleasure into his day. As we talked about other activities, writing kept emerging as a highly valued activity. He had formerly written on the typewriter, but found this impossible due to poor eyesight and weakness in his hands. Since he occasionally wrote notes in session, it was clear that he could write manually, although he did so extremely slowly and with his face nearly on the paper. Over several sessions, we explored the pros and cons of resuming writing, at what was obviously considerable cost and effort. He eventually decided it was worth the trouble and began to write again.

He hunched over the kitchen table in his apartment and laboriously resumed his writing. He would produce one or two pencil-written pages per week. The improvement in his mood was dramatic. Although it was costly in time and effort, he enjoyed the process so much that he found it sufficiently rewarding to continue. On his own initiative, he persuaded his wife to type up what he had written, as she had done in their middle-aged years together. This renewed collaboration seemed to recall happier times for both of them and reestablish a basis for their relationship. The process of writing also led automatically to a life review process for him, which both gave him an enhanced sense of self-worth and provided the two of them with renewed memories of the considerable ups and downs of their lives together, described by John as like the *Days of Wine and Roses*.

While these changes seemed to be wholly positive from John's point of view, and his wife mostly described them as positive for her, subsequent events suggest that she did not find the changes in her husband an unmixed blessing. After a period of a few weeks of missed and rescheduled appointments, I was quite surprised to receive a call from a local nursing home, relaying John's request that I come there to visit him. During this visit, John reported that his wife had checked him into this facility 3 weeks earlier so that she could go visit friends in a mountain community about 200 miles inland. She had told him that she would return in 2 weeks to take him home. She had not returned, and his calls to her friend's house were not being returned. He was, of course, quite distressed and feeling tricked and abandoned.

This change in setting and circumstances required changes in the content of the therapy. His first concern was an attempt to understand what had happened to change his wife's mind and lead her to desert him there. He at first assumed that things had changed after she left, but a review of the move suggested that she had planned not to return. That is, they had been forced to leave their apartment, which was being converted into condominiums, and she had moved most of his belongings to the nursing home and disposed of others. Although there were vague plans of her returning to look for a place, some discussion with the nursing home staff made it clear that she had not arranged for just a 2-week stay. Bewilderment turned to anger at the deception and desertion. After a few weeks of anger, hurt and a desire to see her again became predominant.

He also wanted very much to leave the facility and try to live on his own. We discussed the pros and cons of this for several weeks. He had been very dependent on his wife for several years for basic needs such as cooking, cleaning, and mobility. His ability to walk had apparently declined sharply prior to his wife's departure and had become progressively worse after his admission to the facility. The staff there insisted on his using a wheelchair because of his extremely frail and shaky appearance when he tried to walk with canes. Although he got daily assisted exercise, he continued to weaken in ability to walk, and in a few months he was wheelchair-bound and needed assistance to transfer from bed to wheelchair.

He continued to insist that he could make it on his own in an apartment if some friends could be mobilized to help. He did manage at this point to get local members of the Gambler's Anonymous group to visit and to contact old friends living in Los Angeles. When these friends refused to move him out, and when he discovered how much local apartments cost, he accepted the idea of remaining in the nursing facility. This acceptance seemed to result in reduced anger without an increase in depression, an outcome that both surprised and pleased me.

He also maintained, with minimal encouragement from me, his listening to music and his writing. The nursing and activities staffs both found him refreshing for his intelligence and sense of humor. His main "adjustment" problem was that he hated having roommates and was never paired with anyone who did not annoy him. He dealt with this problem and with the distractions of institutional life by keeping his curtain closed and often leaving his hearing aid turned off.

At this point his writing and our visits became much more focused on life review. He had little to say about his childhood; he had felt lonely and deserted by both parents. His father had been alcoholic and abusive verbally and physically. He had very little to say about his mother. He turned to drinking in his teens and to gambling as soon as he made enough money to gamble with. He had been married before (a fact that had not come out earlier). He had deserted his first wife, who "was not understanding enough." At this point in his life, he also admitted that she had had a lot to put up with. He had cycled in and out of AA in his early adult years and then discovered GA and started a chapter.

He defined his primary problem as the gambling, and his eyes still sparkled when he talked of good gambling trips to Las Vegas and days at the horse races. He moved into higher and higher levels of leadership in GA and enjoyed it even more than gambling. He apparently was perceived as a charismatic leader and even as a philosopher in the organization. He continued to slip periodically. It took him decades to decide to quit drinking. He had gambling sprees every few years. On direct questioning, he revealed that only his disabling stroke had stopped this pattern.

His relationship with his second wife had been easier. They had both shared a drinking problem and then had entered AA together. (It was also news to me that his wife had a history of alcoholism.) They had managed to stay sober more than not, although his wife maintained tranquilizer use indefinitely. She had functioned as his assistant and secretary. Reading between the lines of his story, it was easy to see that he had been clearly dominant and had overshadowed her until his illness. He had controlled their lives together and had probably been very temperamental. He admitted to shouting and verbal abuse. He had found most of her friends "dizzy and dumb." He had no children from either marriage and did not seem to wonder about this. Although he began to realize that taking care of him was almost certainly too much to ask of her, he continued to fantasize that she would return and rescue him from the nursing home. She did, in fact, appear for unexpected visits once or twice a year, but did not take him out of the home.

His renewed connection with GA led to his being invited to an anniversary celebration of the chapter he had founded. He wrote a historical speech. Because his voice was barely audible, a week before the meeting he decided to ask someone else to read the speech while he stood at the podium. Weeks were spent in preparation and in reminiscence of his days with the organization. The event was quite a success from John's point of view.

Having accomplished this, he seem to lapse into a more relaxed state of acceptance. His physical condition declined more, while he seemed to remain emotionally stable, though he tired of reviewing his life. We discussed terminating the therapy visits, a prospect that seemed to trouble John less than it did me. After some discussion of how he would do without continued visits, we gradually reduced the frequency of my visits and finally stopped them.

DISCUSSION

Rapport Building. In bringing a current client's spouse into therapy, issues of the therapist's identification with the spouse often predominate in the early phase of therapy. John was remarkably unconcerned about my being influenced by his wife's perspective. In large part, this lack of concern was likely due to his point of view being so completely merged with hers in the initial sessions. My insistence on getting him to talk about how he saw things also automatically avoided my being seen as either "her therapist" or her ally against him.

The major problem in building rapport with John was simply that of communicating with him. John illustrates in one example many of the potential communication problems due to sensory and expressive disabilities. He was unable to see well, so communication from me had to be explicitly verbal: Head-nodding and facial expression of emotion on my part had to be verbalized. Especially after he was placed in the nursing home, it was necessary to announce my arrival and tell him who it was, because his eyesight was too poor to recognize me. His hearing and speech were also extremely poor, but communication was possible by slowing down, sitting close, and supplementing verbal communication with written when a specific word or sentence was hard to get across. Clearly, this makes communication slow and difficult; it does not make communication impossible. The demonstration of willingness to make this effort to achieve contact is an important part of establishing rapport with a disabled client.

Techniques in Therapy. The work with John draws on at least three approaches to change: Lewinsohn's pleasant events theory (Lewinsohn, & MacPhillamy, 1974; Lewinsohn et al., 1978), rehabilitative counseling with the disabled, and life review. With pleasant events theory, as with any behaviorally oriented therapy, the initial step is to involve the client in setting goals for therapy. In fact, as already noted, it took several sessions to help John rediscover his own point of view and get involved in setting goals. The next step is identification of the pleasant events for this particular individual. In working with physically disabled persons, this step becomes somewhat more complicated in that each activity formerly enjoyed must be assessed as to whether it is still physically possible. In John's case, many such activities were no longer possible and certainly not possible in the same frequency as in his life before disability.

As this assessment is done, an important concept to introduce is the notion of the person's average mood level. Developed in Lewinsohn's "Coping with Depression" classes (Lewinsohn et al., 1978), the concept is simply that everyone's mood fluctuates day by day, but that there is an average level that is modifiable. An important corollary is that change in this average will be gradual, so monitoring of the average mood is used to check progress in therapy, with any increase considered a success, rather than comparing how one feels today with the memory of predepression mood and concluding that no change is taking place. For a person as disabled as John, it is critically important to establish early that you realize that life will never be as good as it was before the disability began. On the other hand, the therapist can establish the realistic goal of improving the mood that results from disability plus depression.

While Lewinsohn used extensive paperwork monitoring of these moods and the pleasant events, in most work with older adults, I have found it possible to rely on simpler diaries and verbal reports. Certainly with an individual as disabled as John, the workload of therapy has to be kept light.

With the disabled individual, another modification of this concept is important. There will be a need to give up on some previous activities and, in most cases, recognize that the level of happiness experienced before the disability may no longer be achievable. Instead, the goal becomes to improve mood over what it has been with the combination of disability and depression. The goal becomes improvement rather than attaining past happiness. As is illustrated in John's case, such improvement in mood is quite possible. In fact, John was able to resume more activity,

and put more effort into doing so, than I would have predicted at
the outset of the therapy.

Adjusting these goals and deciding that some activities are no
longer possible takes the therapy into the realm of rehabilitative
counseling and a kind of modified grief work. The opportunity to
talk explicitly about lost abilities is not common in our society,
nor is the opportunity to grieve for these losses. There is a fairly
strong norm for ignoring disability, offering false reassurance to
the disabled, and expecting everyone to talk positively about the
loss of ability (cf. Peters-Golden, 1982). Having some opportunity
to discuss frankly what abilities are gone forever, and to express
anger and/or depression about these losses, is an important step
to true adjustment. The lack of opportunity to express emotion
tends to lead to ruminative thoughts about these emotions, which
in turn prevents normal problem solving. In John's life, the opportunity to talk about what he could not do, and to first be angry
and then sad about these very significant losses, freed him to
think about what he could still do.

Another common source of resistance to change is the disabled
person's perception of the burden that he or she imposes on the
caregiver. The disabled person is generally aware of this burden
and fearful that the caregiver will decide that it is too heavy a load
and will leave. This fear tends to impede communication about
the illness and often about how to make life better for both people. In John's case, this fear kept him intensely aware of his wife's
needs and unable to think about what he could do. Becoming
more aware of his remaining abilities reduced his wife's caregiving workload, a situation that would often be considered an improvement. In this instance, his wife left him.

Therapy fairly often has unexpected and unintended consequences. In this instance, both John and his wife experienced
some considerable improvement in mood after a few months of
therapy and seemed to achieve a new and happier balance in the
relationship. Not long after this, however, his wife put him in a
nursing home and left him. Apparently they had a relationship
that was balanced as long as both felt depressed and helpless. For
his wife, the changes seem to have led to a desire to change her
life completely.

As seen in the case presentation, John's admission to the nursing home led to another crisis in evaluating and accepting his disability. He was also faced with the problem of understanding his wife's departure from his life. Both of these became entwined in a life review process. He developed a better understanding of their relationship, including the awareness that he had been hard on her and had not built up many credits to draw on for caretaking in his old age. He also came to realize that he had been dominant and strong in the relationship and that she would have trouble accepting him as weak and dependent.

He drew great pleasure from his earlier successes in life and his renewal of contacts with people who remembered him and still valued him for his earlier contributions. He became able to accept his life as it had been, with many positives and many negatives, and to appreciate the relationship between his past and where and how his life was ending. In John's case, I am less inclined to interpret this review process in Erikson's term, as a struggle with developmental stages and unfinished business, than to see it in more cognitive terms as a need to achieve a coherent theory to explain why his wife had left and why he was in a nursing home. George Kelly (1955), in his personal constructs theory, relates much of anxiety and distress to the sense of being unable to explain crisis events in life.

In developing an explanation that reinterpreted the events and the history leading up to them, John was able to restore a sense of order and control to his life after it had been seriously disrupted by the crisis of unexpected and unexplained placement in the nursing home.

Gerontological Issues. In working with John, the major issues centered on disability and rehabilitation rather than age-related differences as such. In fact, the tendency to view the changes as related to age was one of the perceptions that I worked to change in helping John define his problems. His disabilities were related to strokes and other cardiovascular disease rather than to normal aging. Recognizing this distinction provided a different basis for problem solving and a different outlook for the future. Clearly he was going to get older, but he was not necessarily going to become progressively more disabled. The distinction also gave his dysfunctions greater specificity: He had particular disabilities for particular reasons. Reframing the causality in this way also immediately raises the questions of what abilities he had left, and whether existing abilities could be increased with practice.

The communication issues with John are similarly seen as specific to disability rather than age. Not all elderly have visual and hearing impairment, although many do. Therapists working with the elderly will need greater skill in communicating with the visually and hearing impaired of all ages. The problem is a gerontological one in that the proportion of older adults with such problems is higher, and so one cannot work with the elderly without experiencing such problems. Considering the problem to be aging-related leads to two erroneous conclusions: that all older people will have such problems and that the issue never arises with younger clients.

Issues of caregiving and later-life marriage clearly arise in this example. As is more common in later life, the balance of their relationship had been completely altered by his illness: An external event beyond their control reshaped the role each could play, and had to play, in the relationship. Their relationship was not well suited to adapting to such a change. A stormy marriage, based in part on John's being in a dominant and commanding role and leading or caring for his wife, was forced into a pattern of his wife having to care for him as a disabled, very frail, depressed, and uncertain man.

The change of setting during the therapy, from community-based clinic office visits to nursing home visits at his bedside, illustrates one of the prime service principles of working with the elderly. If therapy is to continue, clients who can no longer come to the office must be visited wherever they are. The disjuncture between community life and nursing home life for the older adult is dramatic in and of itself, but is often made even worse by separation from all social contacts that existed prior to the move.

Family members fairly often stay involved with the institutionalized older adult. Friends very rarely do. In addition, most community-based services are set up to serve people while they reside in the community, but terminate services when the client is admitted to nursing home care. For several months after his placement, I was John's only visitor and only continuity with his previous life. Fortunately he had enough contacts outside that he eventually was able to find friends who would visit, but this process took several weeks and considerable encouragement from me.

Relationship Issues. My initial reaction to John was a sense of being overwhelmed by his problems and a sense of helplessness stimulated by his frail appearance. Guided by cognitive-behavioral theory, which argues that anyone is capable of some change, I forged ahead with the work and was quite surprised by his response to therapy. As I became better acquainted with him, I was very impressed by his intelligence, humor, and generally philosophical acceptance of what life had to offer him at present. His response to me was generally positive and mostly role specific. That is, I think he liked me and appreciated the constancy of my visits, but I never had a feeling that he developed a deeper or transferential relationship to me.

On the other hand, over the early months I came to associate John with my father, who had also been quite physically frail toward the end of his life. This positive countertransference became a problem for me at two points in the therapy: when his wife checked him into the nursing home and when it came time to terminate therapy. In the first instance, I found that my feelings toward his wife were more angry and negative than John's feelings were. I had to be alert constantly to the danger of imposing my feelings on him. John was surprised and hurt, and he longed to see his wife again. I was angry with her and wanted to give her a piece of my mind. This latter was my problem, however, and not John's.

After his speech to the Gambler's Anonymous meeting, our visits lost a sense of direction. After more time had passed, I began to sense that he seemed to be wondering why I was still coming. In general, I am not prone to extend therapy indefinitely; however, I found myself very reluctant to stop seeing John. After some discussion of this reluctance with other team members, I came to realize that I was more attached to him than was appropriate to the situation and that, in some ways, I was trying to make up for my infrequent visits to my father, who had been in a nursing home during my graduate school years. Soon after this realization, we were able to terminate therapy with mutual good feeling.

Summary. John is an excellent example of the potential for change in an older disabled person, who was quite frail and appeared even more so. He was able to improve his mood substantially and achieve an emotional adjustment during a time when his life changed significantly for the worse. He was also able to renew an interest in activities that were quite effortful but also quite rewarding for him.

CHAPTER FOUR

Frances:
Generalized Anxiety

One of the first older clients that I saw, Frances was in her early 70s when I met her. She sought therapy because of recurring dreams, constant worrying, and occasional episodes of feeling confused and disoriented and unable to do anything at all. She had known psychologists in the past, having retired from state civil service work in juvenile corrections. Some of her children and grandchildren had seen therapists and had been helped by them.

Her description of her problems sounded very much like an anxiety disorder, and she assured me that she had no physical problems. I started with progressive relaxation training, which she took to very readily and practiced daily with some immediate improvement in her symptoms. We also began trying to pinpoint when the anxiety episodes tended to occur.

At this point, she knew that her sleep was disturbed by dreams, but was unable to recall the content of the dreams. I tried then to get her to keep records of when the episodes occurred, what was happening before, and what happened after they stopped. She virtually never came in with written records completed, but did adopt the structure suggested for describing times when she felt anxious. For several weeks no very clear pattern emerged. Many episodes, but not most, seemed to occur after interactions with other people, especially phone calls from family, yet others would just happen as she worked around the house, talked to her cats, or listened to the radio.

We also spent part of each session talking about psychologists that we both knew, or she might share interactions with neighbors that she thought were particularly amusing. Sometimes she would tell stories about "her girls," the young offenders she had worked with for several decades who had nicknamed her "the Owl" because she never missed anything when they were trying to pull tricks on her. Aside from being intrinsically interesting, these stories helped to bolster her self-esteem and remind her of times when she had been very competent and in control.

After several weeks and gradual improvement in her average level of anxiety, Frances got a telephone call from a former daughter-in-law that upset her greatly. In relating this call to me, she revealed that her granddaughter, Ellen, had run away from home (where she had lived with this daughter-in-law) a couple of years earlier and had not been heard from since. Frances was very worried about this girl, who would have been about 15, and was certain that the girl's mother knew more about the disappearance than she was telling.

It developed that she was, understandably, very preoccupied with her missing granddaughter and that most of her anxiety was started by conversations that reminded her of Ellen, sometimes quite indirectly. She listened to talk radio a lot, and any mention of runaways or calls from runaways would lead to anxious hours. Over the next several weeks, she began to remember and report her disturbing dreams, which were almost entirely about what might be happening to Ellen.

While continuing the relaxation strategies, we focused the next several sessions on talking about Ellen. Frances talked about her fears and worries about where Ellen was now, literally uncertain whether she would be safer alive or dead. She had much to say about the parenting failures of both the daughter-in-law and her own son. They were divorced after a very stormy relationship; at this point, the son was an out-of-control alcoholic who was in danger of dying from liver disease in his 40s. She also reviewed her own relationship with her grandchildren over and over to see what she might have done that would have encouraged the girl to run to her.

After several weeks of this talk, she came to the conclusion that Ellen was probably alive and safe and would "make herself known" when she turned 18 and could not be forced to return to her parents. This decision alleviated her anxiety considerably, although she continued to have bouts of anxiety and despair.

In talking about Ellen's relationship with her mother and reviewing her own performance as a grandmother, Frances also
talked about her own early life. She was an illegitimate child and
had been left by her mother with friends of the family, who had
taken her in and provided for her and "raised me right," but had
not been affectionate people. In fact, it seemed clear to Frances
that they acted out of a sense of moral obligation as good church
people, but felt somewhat put upon to have to be raising a child
again. She felt that both her sense of abandonment and the lack of
active affection from her foster parents had affected her as both
parent and grandparent.

There was clearly a sense of wistful incompletion about her
own mother. In order to help her express some of these feelings, I
set up a role play with her mother represented by an empty chair.
With considerable prompting from me (to keep speaking, not
about what to say) she told "her mother" many of the things that
she had not fully articulated to herself about why she had been
left and her feelings of loss, anger, and so on. Although there was
a clear sense of her doing this exercise mostly to humor me, she
seemed to become involved in it. There was a further reduction in
anxiety after this.

After this point, we discussed her progress to date and talked
about reducing the frequency of sessions and terminating soon. A
couple of months later she missed some sessions and I got a call
from her son, explaining that she had been found unconscious
one night and had been taken to the hospital, where she was diagnosed as having diabetes. Unfortunately, the toes on one foot
had become gangrenous and had to be amputated.

When she returned to therapy, we talked about her surgery, her
reaction to the diagnosis, and her feelings of resistance to complying with medication and diet regimens. I was quite distressed to
learn at this point that she had not seen a doctor in years, even
though she had been feeling physically uncomfortable and had
known that she had an infection or something in her foot. It also
developed that much of what we had interpreted as residual anxiety cleared up when her blood sugar was under control. The doctor also diagnosed a previously unrecognized visual impairment
(diabetic retinopathy).

The combination of being confronted with her physical frailty and her 75th birthday brought home to Frances her personal mortality. In some ways, she had been so preoccupied with her granddaughter that her own physical limitations and approaching death had been ignored. Over several months of home visits, which took place sitting under a tree in her yard because she did not want me to see her housekeeping, we moved through stages of denial, anger, bargaining, and depression to acceptance. Along the way, we talked of her divorce, her pride in her work, and her feeling of having neglected her children (all of whom had, in fact, significant emotional or relationship problems and most of whom were alienated from her).

This phase of therapy terminated soon after she accepted her mortality. This was 8 years ago as I write this, and Frances is still living and in relatively good spirits, although both her mobility and her vision are considerably more limited than at that time.

DISCUSSION

Rapport Building. Frances was already prepared for psychotherapy and very positive about psychologists, based on her work experience in corrections. She was not, however, an older version of the YAVIS (Young Attractive Verbal Intelligent Successful) client. She had a high school education, had enjoyed a long career as a frontline worker in juvenile corrections, and was a longtime resident of the poorest neighborhood in the small city in which she lived. Our conversations often included her commentary on local gang activity, someone trying her door late at night, or gunfire across her backyard.

Techniques in Therapy. Frances's therapy proceeded in unusually well-defined separate stages. In the first phase, we pursued a very cognitive-behavioral course, using relaxation training to reduce the intensity of her anxiety attacks and exploring for patterns in her anxiety. Following personal constructs theory (Kelly, 1955) and George Kelly's principle that anxiety is largely the result of uncertainty, it seemed to me that understanding the source and the pattern of her anxiety would make the attacks themselves more predictable and less anxiety-arousing. Both of these worked to a degree. She used relaxation training quite well and did experience a further reduction in anxiety when we discovered the relationship of the attacks to concern for her missing granddaughter.

The missing granddaughter served as the trigger for a new phase of the therapy, based on using a family systems perspective in the individual therapy. As she talked about her granddaughter, Frances's family history and her own sense of rejection in her family of origin emerged and assumed a central role in the therapy. Note that there was both identification and contrast in her sense of relationship to her granddaughter. She identified with the young woman in the sense of knowing what it felt like to grow up without feeling loved and nurtured. On the other hand, there was a sense of the granddaughter's having run away from a relatively safe home into a dangerous world, whereas she (Frances) had been abandoned by her mother and could not imagine anyone with a mother giving that up.

This sense of conflict within herself, as well as a strong sense of unfinished business with her mother, further fed her anxiety. Talking her way through the conflict helped her see in what ways she and Ellen were similar and different. The chance to "talk with" her mother, using the empty chair technique borrowed from gestalt therapy, helped her to complete unfinished conversations with her mother in a more concrete and emotionally evocative manner than simply talking about her mother (cf. Polster & Polster, 1973). Again, there was further reduction in anxiety.

With the discovery of her illness, Frances began to feel old and close to death. As described, we went through a series of sessions preparing her for dying that very closely followed Kübler-Ross's (1969) stages and principles for accepting the coming of death. As has occurred in most such cases in my work with older adults, there was also a spontaneous life review. At the end of this work, not only did she feel better emotionally but her health also improved. While it is perhaps doubtful that the upswing in her health was related to the reduction in anxiety, it is ironic that one of the most technically perfect preparation-for-dying therapies in my career was with someone who has lived more than a decade past the completion of the counseling. One lesson to be learned from this is that being prepared for death may also prepare one for living with chronic, progressive illness and its constant reminder of physical frailty and approaching death.

Gerontological Issues. Occurring at an early point in my career, the dramatic appearance of Frances's illness after a few months in therapy was a pivotal event in focusing my attention on the inter-relationship between medical and psychological factors in helping older adults. While I was intellectually aware of the increasing in-terrelationship of physical and psychological factors that comes with aging, I had not really translated these concerns into daily clinical practice. Instead, as I believe is fairly typical of young psychosocially trained professionals, I tended to deal with the physical/medical side of clients' lives by ignoring it as much as possible.

In Frances's case, it seemed to me that two problems resulted from this narrow focus on psychological issues: First, it had sim-ply not occurred to me to ask about her medical diagnoses and the frequency of contact with physicians; I simply accepted her statement that she had no physical problems. She had been grad-ually getting worse in her walking, but I had not actually noticed this until after the fact. Since that time, I have become more con-cerned with making certain that clients have physicians and have seen them recently. I have also made it a practice to be certain to encourage clients to speak to a physician about any physical or functional change that occurs during the course of therapy.

Second, it seemed quite likely that some of her apparent anxiety was due to the diabetes. This likelihood left me in the somewhat embarrassing spot of having treated physically based symptoms with psychological interventions. Again, it is one thing to be aware of these issues in the abstract, and another to put that awareness into practice. One can further note that Frances herself was both quite psychologically minded and also intent on avoid-ing physicians as much as possible. Nonetheless, her case illus-trates quite well the problems inherent in taking too narrow a view of the older adult.

On a more positive note, Frances also illustrates one way in which an essentially completely emotion-focused intervention can help a physically frail older person with a progressive illness feel better and achieve a better quality of life. All too often within aging services, physical frailty is seen as requiring only medical and casework interventions, and the role of emotional intervention is overlooked.

She also illustrates, in a different way from other cases in this volume, the unpredictability of death. Frances was looking extremely physically frail and was feelings very physically weak when we began to talk about preparing for her death. She has gone on to live 10 years since that time with increasing physical frailty. In the earlier years of my work with the elderly, I was inclined to associate physical frailty and multiple chronic illness with nearness to death. A decade of experience has taught me that one can live a long time close to death. This lesson is probably emotionally more difficult to absorb than the death of clients.

Frances and her dysfunctional family also serve as an important cautionary note to our preoccupation with keeping older people involved with their families. Frances's family relationships were mostly dysfunctional, and contact with family members tended to be distressing rather than supportive. When family members got in touch, it was often because they were looking for help from her. While there clearly are loving and supportive families, we need to recall that abusive, violent, and otherwise dysfunctional families also grow old together.

Relationship Issues. Between the alienation from her own family and the similarity in age between myself and her son, it is not surprising that Frances was inclined to identify me as a good son who was helpful to her. This role generalized to some extent to other family members, who were also inclined to put me in the role of the responsible son. Her own son, living with her while recovering from alcoholism, would often call me and ask that I try to get her to see a doctor or agree to surgery when she was balking. On the whole, the positive transference on her part tended to help the progress of therapy. We were able at times to discuss how our professional relationship was different from family or other personal ties.

On my side, for several months afterward I felt rather guilty about not recognizing her illness. While I was largely able to channel these feelings into learning more about health psychology, I also felt restrained from being confrontive with her for a while. Fortunately I recognized this feeling, knew what was going on, and was able to talk it out with other team members so that the therapy was not obstructed.

In a more general way, I liked Frances very much. She was sharp, insightful, and funny, and she had considerable wisdom gleaned from a lifetime of contact with people of all kinds. It was Frances who once observed, after a discussion group about aging, that growing older had been easier for her because she had always been "plain," whereas more attractive women had to struggle more with the changes that aging brings in physical appearance. Liking her also made it sad and often painful to see her physical decline over the next several years as she lost her eyesight and became more and more limited in her ability to walk. The last time I saw her, getting around in her own living room was difficult. Watching older people, whom you like and know with the intimacy of therapy, become more and more disabled is one of the most difficult aspects of psychotherapy with the elderly.

Summary. Frances illustrates a number of important lessons in working with anxious older adults. Her therapy included both immediate, present-oriented interventions and some need to review her life and resolve unfinished business with her own mother. She also underlines the important lesson of the coexistence of medical and psychological problems in older adults. With older clients, the psychotherapist will have to be more actively concerned with clients' health problems while focusing on assisting with psychological issues.

CHAPTER FIVE

Elaine and Warren:
Caregiving Issues

The first contact with Elaine and Warren came with her seeking help because she felt overwhelmed and frustrated in helping care for Warren. He had Chronic Obstructive Pulmonary Disease (COPD) and was supposed to be on oxygen 24 hours a day, but usually used it considerably less. She was seen individually a few times by another member of the Senior Outreach team. Warren was referred to me when they were disagreeing about the wisdom of his wanting to travel out-of-state to see family.

Although she had been seeking help to reduce her stress, her sessions had been split between concern over his not following his medical treatment carefully and frustration that he was not doing as much around the house as he used to, causing the additional work to fall on her. Their mutual denial of the seriousness of his condition was such that she had him taking down window screens, and both of them were surprised that he became short of breath and was fatigued for several days afterward. On another early occasion they had their house repainted, another decision that debilitated him for a few days.

Warren was a pleasant, soft-spoken man in his late 70s. He brought with him, but did not use, a small portable oxygen tank. His breathing was noticeably labored. He admitted to feeling depressed and fatigued much of the time. He was uncertain how much was due to his physical condition and how much was true sadness. He denied feeling any irritation with his wife's demands, asserting that it was "just her way" to be fussy about the house and want things very nice. He recognized that she had trouble accepting his limitations.

In response to my questioning, Warren stated that the doctor had prescribed oxygen 24 hours a day, but he preferred to use it less and, in fact, was using it closer to 6 hours daily. He reluctantly admitted that the doctor had told him that the oxygen would help him feel less tired. Warren equated using the oxygen with being ill and felt that the less he used it, the less ill he was. We discussed the logic of this and he admitted, without much conviction, that the illness was there and the oxygen was a treatment that would help him feel better, but he was not using it. After some bargaining, we started a behavioral contract for more use of the oxygen each day, targeting some early evening hours when he felt especially bad.

When we discussed his trip to Utah, his expectations did seem unrealistic. The concern was not so much the trip itself, but his expectation of driving long hours each day and going on a lengthy fishing trip once he got there. With a joint session, they negotiated for somewhat more realistic plans and went on the trip.

After their return, Warren and Elaine continued to be seen individually, working on medical treatment adherence issues with him and lower expectations in her case. Her therapist focused on acceptance of his illness and of the consequent changes that might come into their lives. Elaine was a compulsive housekeeper, and both of them disliked spending money to get others to help. The result was that she continued her own high demands for her work while also taking on his jobs around the house.

This takeover included gardening and an attempt to mow the lawn, which almost resulted in a stroke for her. At about this time, we discovered her previous history of heart disease and strokes. There was also an interesting family history that partly accounted for her reluctance to travel back to see the family. She and Warren had been married somewhat more than 15 years, each for the second time. They had previously been in-laws (their late spouses were brother and sister) and had comforted each other when their respective spouses had died within the space of a couple of years. This had caused some stir within the family, and his children had trouble accepting Aunt Elaine as a stepmother. Her previous husband had died quickly and unexpectedly of a heart attack, and she could not face the possibility that Warren would also become ill and die.

After a previous appointment ended early, I stepped into the waiting room one day to see Warren with blue-gray skin, drawing deep breaths. He returned fairly rapidly to normal, but through some questioning (to which our secretary was more responsive than were they) we determined that this happened often, because they parked a couple of blocks away rather than using the handicapped parking at the door. At our insistence we began home visits at this point. Prompted by this observation, we questioned them more closely and found that they were not pleased with their medical care, and in particular thought that the doctor was underestimating recent changes in Warren's condition, including his feeling that his lungs were blocked in some way.

Considering that this was coming from two people who were characterized by denial, we were quite concerned and suggested that they either go back to the doctor and discuss their concerns more assertively or seek a second opinion. They followed through on the latter suggestion, and in a few weeks Warren was diagnosed with lung cancer, had surgery, and was informed that there was no further treatment. He was discharged home in a hospital bed, and Elaine's caregiving burden increased significantly. There was a clear implication that Warren would die from this illness, but no indication of how long he would live with it. Unfortunately, at about this same time, her therapist became ill and was off work for several months. I continued seeing both of them at home.

Initially, their reaction was primarily one of anger at the first physician. Elaine was also quite angry at some of the hospital and home health social workers, whom she felt had promised more than the couple had received in services. They were very angry with one young man in particular, who had explained home equity conversion to them as a way of getting funds for more care. They both perceived this as a callous attempt to take their house away from them. Her stress level was so intense, and she was so confused about the situation, that I intervened directly and talked with different caseworkers to clarify the situation as much as I could. This resulted in less confusion and some reduction in anger and anxiety, but no real change in service levels. They were getting all they were entitled to and, in fact, had been enrolled in a new demonstration program, which had given them more weeks of home care than Medicare would normally fund.

Elaine also became concerned about her mental functioning at this point. A psychology intern assigned to our program tested her and found some focal memory losses that were not great, and an assessment that suggested that she perceived more memory problems than she had. Many of her blocks in mental functioning were anxiety-related and greatly increased by now having total responsibility for not only the house but also Warren's home health care.

I made it a point to stop and talk to Warren every week for a few minutes, even though he was at first too weak to talk clearly or even to listen for more than a few sentences. He would nod or shake his head appropriately and squeeze my hand at times. When he did recover, he was very philosophical about his illness and the surgery, while acknowledging some anger at the first physician. He expressed a strong religious conviction that there was always hope and he had confidence in a miracle that would bring him to recovery.

For a while we met together in their living room, with Elaine and me sitting in chairs by his hospital bed. Warren occasionally dozed off during meetings, and Elaine and I would continue. These sessions focused on the exact nature of his cancer, what was left, what the doctors had told them. They expressed considerable anger and disappointment at what had happened. We discussed Elaine's need to "keep everything perfect" and together worked out specific things she would let slide (e.g., not planting a garden this year, not doing the special Easter baking).

They gradually decided to hire a neighbor to do the lawn and got housekeeping assistance as well. Neighbors and church members would visit and let Elaine get out for a while. Her chronic heart problems and hypertension were showing signs of worsening in response to stress, and a chronic neck arthritis was also worsening. She was requiring more doctor visits and had to use much of her "respite" time for her own medical treatment.

Since neither of them would admit to his getting worse, or mention the subject of death in the other's presence, I began dividing visits into her time and his time and talking to them in different rooms. Both expressed great concern about not upsetting the other, and, in fact, being very positive with one another had been a solid rule in their relationship from the beginning. They saw themselves as hard workers and as copers who didn't let anything get them down. To act differently would be a betrayal.

She was keenly aware of the possibility of his death coming soon. Part of her anger about the service programs was that she had been told he would get hospice care, but then he didn't qualify because the physicians could not give a definite prognosis of less than 6 months to live. She felt certain he would die sooner and actually expressed surprise that he was still alive. She had numerous concerns about his death. She had never been alone for long in her entire life and was completely unprepared emotionally for the loneliness of widowhood. Warren's illness was reminding her of her first husband's death, and it was clear to me that she had not completed grieving for that husband and was starting to reexperience some of those feelings now. She was very worried about Warren's will and had some concrete and apparently realistic concerns about what his children would do with the house and the estate if he died without a will. It was clear that she was physically and emotionally exhausted by the work of caring for Warren and unable to express any feelings about this.

For weeks we went over this same content again and again while she gradually became able to express her feelings in a low-key manner. She gained renewed commitment to the therapeutic process when she had a fugue experience one week. After a particularly trying day, she suddenly found herself in the car, driving away from home with no destination in mind. She pulled into a shopping center parking lot and sat there for a couple of hours before she could make herself return.

This experience frightened both of them considerably. She was made keenly aware of how much stress she was under. It brought to the surface his fears that she would decide to leave him because of the burden of caring for him. She also acknowledged for the first time that he was sometimes negative and critical about her care. We were able to talk this through, and she reassured him of her ongoing love and commitment to caring for him. I reassured her that she could prevent future episodes by monitoring her stress better and taking short breaks before she got to the point that she would take unconscious breaks.

The incident also made it clear to me that their needs were different and that I was more allied with her than with Warren. We brought in another therapist, explaining that we felt they each needed someone to talk with and that Warren's original therapist could not return due to health reasons.

Working alone, she was able to talk more about how demanding he was and his criticism of her. She was more open about the stress she was under and revealed being keenly aware of how the physical work of caring for him worsened her own chronic conditions. At one point, she had to postpone until after his death surgery on her neck that would have decreased pain and increased her range of motion. We also discussed how his hope for a miracle prevented her from talking with him about the will and other concrete financial plans for herself. Much of this work was simply listening and being aware that I was the only person she could talk to this way. All of her family and friends shared the optimism and "stiff upper lip" philosophy, whereas I encouraged her to acknowledge the negative possibilities and express her feelings about them.

The other therapist was able to talk with Warren and get into some of his concerns about Elaine and explore his awareness of the possibility of dying. He was able to acknowledge that the doctors expected him to die. Over several sessions, and without challenging his faith that a miracle might intervene, she was able to have him acknowledge the possibility of death and the need to make some plans with Elaine.

We had a conjoint session in which Elaine was able to discuss the need for a will and the kind of changes that would help her. To Elaine's surprise he was already well aware of the problems with his children and very willing to make some appropriate changes to protect her. They were able to acknowledge together, albeit briefly and without much expressed emotion, that there was a possibility that he would die within the next year or so.

After this her concerns were largely with the day-to-day problems of caregiving: oxygen tanks not getting delivered on time, changes in home health nursing staff, arguments with various elements of their formal support network, being surprised by various programs ending services that she needed, because they had reached their quota of care. She was able to express appropriate anger at this situation. She thought it was ridiculous that people set timetables on providing care that had nothing to do with patient need and she could not understand why she got the most care when she had needed it least, which was immediately after he left the hospital.

It became obvious after a few months that part of her method of sustaining herself was through the idea that caregiving was going to be limited. She began to interpret the doctor's statement that Warren had about a year as a guarantee that the hard work of personal care nursing for her husband would last only a year. As the end of that year neared and Warren seemed to stabilize, she began to exhibit increasing signs of distress.

Elaine reluctantly began to describe her feeling that it had to end soon and her fears about being able to maintain in the long run. We were able to gradually separate her need to see an end to this arduous work from any guilt-inducing desire that Warren die soon. This line of conversation also allowed us to talk about what she needed to do differently if, in fact, he were to live for a few more years. She slowly began to accept the need to think about these changes and what she would have to do to take care of herself.

Throughout these discussions, she was unable to form any idea in advance of what her life as a widow would be like. She had married the first time to leave her parents' home and had scarcely been alone between her first husband and Warren. She had no image of living alone and no desire whatsoever to do so. We talked about the need to think ahead, and she did talk to a few friends who were widows, but still found herself totally unable to imagine living that way.

While we were discussing these issues from session to session, one night Warren began choking, was rushed to the hospital by ambulance, and died a couple of weeks later. Family and friends came in for support. Elaine called in for therapy a couple of months later.

She was a changed woman. She seemed more relaxed, smiled easily, and looked several years younger. She was grieving for Warren and having some problems readjusting to widowed life, but these problems were considerably easier than caring for her husband in the last years of his life. We had a few sessions, rather

widely spaced over a few months. She continued to have problems making up her mind and especially struggled over plans to
visit her daughter in the Midwest and the question of whether she
wanted to live near her daughter. She felt she should, but she and
her daughter were both opinionated and headstrong, and Elaine
was wanting to control her own life. She was also rediscovering
friends and church connections that she had almost forgotten. She
attended grieving classes at the mortuary that had handled the
funeral and also attended some through the Senior Outreach
program, where she became friends with another class member. She gradually came in less and less often and terminated
therapy successfully.

DISCUSSION

Rapport Building. Establishing rapport with Elaine and Warren
was remarkably easy, given their background. Both were well
past 70 years old, had grown up in small Western towns, were
high school educated, and were working-class people with a
strong conviction that optimism and hard work would solve life's
problems. This is hardly a portrait of psychologically minded
people who would be prime candidates for psychotherapy. In
spite of this, they were receptive to the idea that they needed help
and willing to consider all the input we had for them.

Our input was often contrary to their lifelong convictions: We
were, after all, challenging their denial of illness; encouraging
them to accept the diagnosis and learn to live with disability; and
encouraging them to look on the negative side of their lives and
express fear, anxiety, and depression. Further, we were telling
them that doing these things was the way to feel better! While
sensible within a psychological worldview, these ideas are clearly
not obvious from other points of view.

Their willingness to work with us and give our way of doing
things a try is based on realities of late life often overlooked by
those who assume that people like Elaine and Warren will be un-
suited for or unwilling to pursue therapy. The problems of later
life are often sufficiently overwhelming that people are ready to
try anything. They also have often overwhelmed lifelong coping

strategies and have left the older client willing to change long-term patterns of handling problems. With a body that is refusing to work right, death approaching, and the demands of caregiving overwhelming the ability to keep life going as usual, the most resistant potential client can be highly motivated for change.

Techniques in Therapy. The earlier phase of work with Elaine and Warren focused largely on their acceptance of the illness and the development of realistic expectations for themselves in continuing their lives. In the beginning, they were virtually textbook examples of denial and its effect on illness. Both were denying his illness and expecting too much from his now-disabled body. The result was frequent exhaustion and relapses. It was physically dangerous for Warren to avoiding the use of oxygen and continue to do demanding household tasks. So was coming to the office for therapy, hence the change to home visits. Continually examining both the logic of what they were doing and the consequences of their actions in a supportive atmosphere helped them to gradually shift to more realistic levels of activity. The supportive atmosphere was an important part of this change: Being psychotherapy-oriented, we were not in a hurry for them to change and we conveyed understanding and sympathy for the difficulty of giving up a long life of being active, in control, and able to overcome every obstacle that arose.

After the discovery of his cancer, the work with Warren focused on preparation for dying, but was limited by both his extreme physical frailty and his strong religious conviction that a miracle would preserve his life. Out of concern for his psychological well-being and the need for communication between the two of them, we pushed only to the extent of making certain he understood that the physicians thought he would die soon. Failure to acknowledge that fact would have seemed like unhealthy denial and would have blocked further communication between the couple. On the other hand, we had no desire to challenge his religious conviction that the doctors would be proved wrong. He was quite willing to make contingency plans with Elaine and to talk with her about the possibility of his death.

Her work was largely anticipatory grieving for her husband and coping with the day-to-day strain of caring for him. The grief work was mostly listening and encouraging this very private and compulsively strong woman to talk about her fears, depression, and fantasies about the future. As we have found in other cases, Elaine was nearly equally balanced between the fear of losing Warren and the fear that he would continue to live and this overwhelming situation would go on for years. Also, much of the grief work was actually focused on grieving the loss of her first husband, who had died quite suddenly and whose death she had coped with by using denial and her "stiff upper lip, life must go on" philosophy. At this point, she was more able to acknowledge the feelings of shock and loss for her first husband.

With these feelings expressed, she moved quite naturally into a review of her relationship with Warren. Almost entirely positive, their relationship had been built on mutual strengths that were mutually reinforcing. The surprise of their extended-blended family at their marriage had served to isolate them in an "us against the world" relationship. There was, however, clearly no historical basis for coping with irresolvable adversity. They had never before met problems they could not solve. They also had no historical basis for taking care of one another; they were strong people who did not need to be taken care of. This life review also led to her realization of having never been alone and having no desire to be a widow with limited prospects of remarriage.

As a caregiver, Elaine had a nearly perfect formula for high distress. She was herself physically frail and in chronic pain. She had a mild, nonprogressive cognitive impairment due to her stroke. She was obsessive-compulsive in personality style: She worried constantly, she wanted everything perfect and on time, she had considerable trouble accepting alterations in lifelong patterns, and she wanted the system of services available to her to make sense. In addition to trying to do too much herself, possessing these qualities meant that it was hard both to give up having a neatly trimmed lawn and to hire someone to mow the lawn. Every slipup in home-care schedules, such as workers being late for appointments and unannounced changes in who was coming out, were very upsetting for her.

The irrationality of policy surrounding home care was extremely frustrating for her: Warren was clearly dying, why couldn't they have hospice care? Why couldn't they decide when they needed help, instead of having to accept more hours than they needed when he was bedbound and unconscious and getting fewer hours as his condition worsened and their postdischarge time increased?

Fortunately, much of the earlier work, on giving up highly stressful tasks and lowering expectations, was generalizable to this period of her life, and Elaine learned to manage her stress reasonably well. The couple's work focused on communication. For this couple, talking about the possibility of his death, their feelings, and the need to settle certain issues was a major change from their usual historical pattern of optimistic problem-solving communication. With individual preparation and rehearsal, they were able to open up enough to share important feelings and make some essential plans for Elaine's future.

Gerontological Issues. Elaine and Warren bring to life the gerontological adage that the old must be understood and served within a biopsychosocial framework. Although they were seeing us for psychological problems and issues, much of their early therapy focused on medical issues and could be understood within the framework of health psychology. At a key point in their lives, they presented us with physical symptoms that they felt needed more attention, and we explored various options with them. After verifying with them that they had talked with their current physician and were dissatisfied with the response, we pointed out that they had the right to a second opinion.

On the social services side, after hospital discharge they were extremely upset with the kind of services they had versus what they felt they needed, and were also dismayed at the cost of these services. Our ability to check out these services in the aging services and home health services networks was important for them. In this instance, we did not find new services but instead informed Elaine that they had, in fact, gotten the best service package available and that some of the caseworkers involved had actually gone to special trouble to arrange unusually good deals for them. We also sympathized with her feeling that the best available was not good enough. It is also an instructive insight into the services system that Elaine and Warren were seen as complaining, angry, and unreasonable people, while they saw themselves as reasonable longtime taxpayers who had always assumed that adequate services were available in the unlikely event that they would ever need them.

The ability to function as both case manager and psychotherapist can be an essential part of serving older adults (cf. Knight, 1986, 1989; Sherman, 1981; Zarit, 1980). In this instance, Elaine would not have been served well by another case manager who could not have arranged better services, nor would the exploration of her feelings about the situation have been helpful without the reality check on what had actually happened and what actually was available. The combination of being able to recheck the casework that had been done and being able to talk with her about the services and her feelings about the services was effective in reducing her distress.

Some therapists argue that such direct intervention is always inappropriate and will increase client dependency; however, I have never found that taking appropriate direct action during psychotherapy has either generated uncontrollable dependency in the client or diminished my status as the psychotherapist. I also see such arguments as rationalizations on the part of professionals who are unwilling to take necessary steps to help clients as needed. At the same time, I view providing such direct services as an inappropriate and unhelpful response when listening and emotionally oriented work are truly needed. Working with older clients constantly poses the question of which approach is more beneficial.

Working with Elaine and Warren as a couple, and for a while seeing each of them as individuals, points out the different actions that might be taken had only one of them been the client, versus what is suggested when working with the couple from a systems perspective. As Margolin (1982) argued some years ago, the choice to conceptualize a case as an individual therapy case instead of a couple's (or family) case is a basic choice with profound ethical implications. Had I been working with Warren individually, my intervention would likely have been more limited and less continuous because of his physical frailty and religious convictions. Any interactions with Elaine would likely have emphasized Warren's need for her and encouraged her to continue caring for him. This well-intended work on my part would have

increased her burden and would likely have resulted in her running away from the situation or pushing herself until she became
ill. Remember that, given her style of presenting herself, I would
not have known how frail she was.

Individual intervention with Elaine would very likely have
stayed focused on the extent of her distress, her anticipatory grief,
and her need to take care of herself. Such an approach might very
well have encouraged her to put Warren in a nursing home as she
fearfully contemplated an indefinite period of caregiving.

The couple's perspective led us to encourage them to talk with
one another, led to some balancing of their needs in our minds,
and also led to some compromising of needs between the two of
them. Seeing them together made it clear to us how much they
cared for one another. We also conceptualized many of their issues
as problems of the couple as a system, rather than as difficulties one
of them had caused for the other. The compromises clearly involved
prolonging Elaine's stress.

At this juncture, it is not my desire to argue that one or another
approach is better. The experience of having done both individual
and systems-level work points up how very different the intervention can be, depending on who and how many people are defined as "the client." It is just recently that the implications of
these differing perspectives in understanding the elderly, and in
making ethically sound decisions about serving older adults and
their families, have been explored (Bumagin & Hirn, 1990; Carter
& McGoldrick, 1988).

Relationship Issues. To the extent that there were transferential
components in Elaine and Warren's relationship to us, I would describe those as starting after Warren's hospitalization and falling
into the positive grandchild transference category: We were accepted as much younger caring and cared for adults, whose ear-
nest competence was both accepted and indulged. This aspect of
the relationship was generally helpful to the therapy.

On the countertransference side, working with Warren quite
clearly aroused all of the feelings associated with watching someone
become very ill and die. Seeing the changes in his health over a
period of a year made very real the devastating effects of the illness. In my own mind and heart, there was considerable conflict

over how long it made sense for him to live coupled with the knowledge that death comes unexpectedly. It made me sad to see him dying and even sadder to know that he could quite possibly live in this condition for years. These were all *my* feelings. It was equally clear to me that Warren wanted very much to go on living and remain at home.

Elaine's ambivalence about whether she was more fearful of Warren's death or of his continuing life in this condition also aroused strong feelings of confusion and sadness in me. Her all but complete inability to think about her own needs and act to take care of herself could be frustrating. At the same time, some decisions (e.g., to postpone her neck surgery) seemed dictated by realistic considerations.

The stark reality of their problems aroused feelings of sadness and feelings of helplessness in me as the therapist; at the same time, to write them off as beyond help seemed to me neither kind nor accurate. They seemed to clearly benefit from our therapeutic conversations. The sadness, helplessness, and frustration then came to be seen as problems of mine that needed to be addressed as I thought about the case and talked about it in team meetings. The ability to express these feelings with other clinicians, and stay focused on our therapeutic goals and progress toward them, helped make it possible to stay involved with this couple as they faced death.

This history with both of them also meant that Elaine's marked improvement after Warren's death was met with mixed feelings on my part. Somewhat prepared for it by experience with other women I had known who became widows while in therapy, I was happy for Elaine but also had to contend with my own reaction that she should be showing more grief for Warren. This reaction was clearly part of my countertransference, however, and not part of her therapy.

Summary. Elaine and Warren illustrate the advantages of being able to work within multiple roles when helping older adults: At various times I worked as individual therapist, case manager, therapist to the couple, and a conjoint therapist working with a cotherapist and the couple. The role flexibility is essential; it is also important to recognize when one is so identified with a client that a cotherapist is necessary. This example also illustrates vividly the need to be knowledgeable about and capable of working with a wide range of other helpers in the aging services network, including physicians, home health nurses, hospice eligibility workers, hospital discharge planners, and more. Finally, they demonstrate the interaction of personality issues, couples' relationship history, and long-term coping styles with the strains of illness, caregiving, and death.

CHAPTER SIX

JoAnn:
Grieving for a Lost Husband

JoAnn was referred for therapy by the health educator in charge of programs for the elderly at a local hospital. She had come to one of the hospital's programs to stop smoking, but had dropped out after a couple of sessions. While discussing this with the health educator, she had appeared to be quite depressed. During their conversation, it came out that her husband had been deceased for less than a year. She had picked the class for ending smoking not only as a way of reestablishing control in her life but also as a social outlet, and then had found it harder than expected. With a few calls from the health educator to explain who I was and what the fees would be for our sessions, JoAnn readily accepted a referral to come in and talk for a few sessions.

She was clearly depressed in that first session. Her facial expression was sad and her speech was slow. She was fatigued, had trouble sleeping, was indecisive, had lost weight due to her poor appetite, and had been isolated and inactive since her husband's death. She often thought about dying with a certain degree of longing, but had no intention of killing herself. She was an intelligent and psychologically minded woman in her early 70s who had been a minister in a liberal church that emphasized intellectual values and modern ideas. Her physician had given her a tricyclic antidepressant, but she "didn't believe in them" and took one only when desperate for sleep. We discussed how this was not an effective pattern for taking the antidepressants, and she acknowledged that her doctor had told her the same thing. She still did not want to take the medication. She took medication for a longtime thyroid problem and had been checked recently for serum thyroid level. She had no other health problems. Although she openly acknowledged her depressed feelings and isolation, when I asked what her goals were for therapy, she replied that she would like to have help stopping smoking.

While I generally like to start with the client's formulation of the problem and work from there, this request seemed sufficiently far off the mark that I negotiated further with her. First, I told her that I did not do much work with smoking cessation and thought that she could get everything I could offer through the hospital program, with the advantages of the group setting. We discussed her experience in trying the group: She had dropped out twice, which had attracted the trainer's attention. She described herself as lacking the energy or the decisiveness to follow through on the homework and so on. After some time on this topic, I asked her quite candidly if she really believed that stopping smoking was the major problem she was facing in her life at this moment. She gave a brief, wry chuckle and shook her head saying, "I guess not."

We then talked about strategies for working on her depression. I explained that I would want to hear her talk more about the death of her husband and the times before and after that event. At that point, my working assumption was that her depression would have to do with unresolved grief and with issues of control in her current life. I also pointed out that her current isolation and level of activity would seem like a sure recipe for depression in a person who was used to intellectual stimulation and social contact. She felt that this approach made sense and was worth trying.

Over the next few sessions, she talked openly about how much she missed her husband and would talk easily about how wonderful their relationship had been prior to his illness. Left to herself, she tended to skip over the period when he had been ill and she had been caring for him. Even with prompting from me, she tended to be evasive, giving brief answers about its having been hard for both of them and then changing the subject to times either before the illness or after his death.

This evasiveness seemed quite important, so I persisted in exploring this time, explaining how stressful caregiving often was for people. I also told her I assumed that her husband had been frustrated with the illness and in some pain and must not have been as sweet and loving as she had described him prior to his illness. This introduction was of some help in exploring this period. She admitted that he may have been "a little negative at times." Any reference to her own feelings at that time was countered by her talking about how she owed it to him, and that marriage involved commitment, even in hard times. She would also throw in at times that people in my generation didn't seem to understand this. Rather than getting pulled into any discussion of this point, I simply agreed with her and told her that my conversations with older people had convinced me that she was right, but that such commitment did not mean that people didn't have feelings.

Over six or more sessions, we gradually established that he had been quite negative, having been in pain most of the last 6 months of his life. In fact, he had been fairly constantly critical, angry, and unappreciative of what she was doing. She constantly excused his behavior and refused to admit negative reactions of her own toward his behavior. I then began interjecting the idea that it was possible to be angry with what someone was doing (or had done) without blaming them for doing it and while continuing to love them very much. "It's possible to be irritated at the critical words without disliking the man who spoke them." She gradually admitted having felt "a little bit irritated" with his negative attitude. I later commented on how hard it is to be angry with someone who is dead and whom you miss very much. She teared up and cried briefly for the first time in therapy.

The next few sessions went over this period of time in some detail. This recounting mainly involved emotional work, with each repetition arousing more emotion from JoAnn. There was some additional indication that this period also marked the start of their isolation. Between the task demands of the caregiving, the reluctance of others to witness his progressive decline in the illness, and his negativity toward those who did come, social contacts decreased to nothing quite rapidly. In her grief, she had done nothing to reestablish those contacts and now felt awkward about contacting old friends to whom she had not spoken in years. In many cases, she felt it was clear that she owed them letters or telephone calls.

It also came out that they had moved to Ventura County just shortly before his illness. With persistent (if sporadic and gentle) questioning on my part, she disclosed that it had been his decision to move there from Los Angeles. He had talked her into the move, based on the idea that friends would come to visit often and they could go to Los Angeles frequently. In fact, this had begun to prove untrue even before he became seriously ill. He had not wanted to travel much, and friends had not visited much. (Several clients who had moved into Ventura from neighboring Los Angeles County have commented on Ventura being farther from Los Angeles than Los Angeles is from Ventura). She had been irritated with him about this when they found out he was ill.

With this out in the open, we did a brief review of their relationship, revealing a common pattern of positives and negatives in which the positives generally prevailed. It is often a part of adjusting to widowhood that the negatives need to be acknowledged. This process does not need to emphasize anger and, in fact, is often quite loving in tone. The need is to bring the deceased back into the realm of real humanity and out of the sainthood status that often accompanies unresolved grief and unacknowledged anger at the deceased loved one.

With this work done, JoAnn was more open and more animated in therapy, but still sad and depressed at home. She continued to be isolated, unable to make decisions, fatigued, sleepless, and uninterested in life. We discussed antidepressants again and she started on a different prescription after consulting with our team psychiatrist, who, in turn, made recommendations to her family care physician. Her sleep became more regular and her energy level improved over the next few months as the dose was increased. She experienced a chronic dryness of her mouth which annoyed her considerably.

We began to work on the renewal of contacts with old friends. As we discussed each situation, the history of the friendship, and the sources of her reluctance, she renewed contact with some of these friends. This process was complicated for her by the fact that most of her friends had known her as their pastor and she was used to being in the helper role, rather than feeling weak and being seen as needing help. This was, in fact, a major and recalcitrant problem, and in each instance of renewing contact with friends, stories came up from her past (going back to childhood) of her need to be the helper or the planner or the one in charge of a relationship.

Before a long-delayed visit to her son who lived in San Francisco, she had a dream of being in a car with her son and her husband when the son was a child. In the dream, she became panic-stricken when she realized no one was behind the wheel as they went up and down hills and around curves. This dream became a symbol of her fear of not being in the driver's seat. Although we discussed this pattern at length, the decision was to work around it by setting up the contacts so that she could look as strong as possible, while being willing with selected friends to admit how she was feeling and seek some comfort or limited help.

During this period she reestablished some control in her life by returning to the stop smoking class and being successful at ending this decades-long habit. She also contracted with me to spend a certain amount of time each week sorting through old legal papers and her financial statements. The need to do this was hers; the idea of contracting for small chunks of the job each week, as a way of making it manageable and of knowing she had to report to someone about her progress, was my strategy.

After visiting her son, she decided to explore selling her house and moving closer to him. She felt she was in Ventura by accident and certainly through no plan of her own. She had a cordial, but not especially close relationship with her son and his family. As we explored her expectations of moving closer to him, she did not expect very frequent contact with the family. In her view, they had their own lives and were quite busy.

We discussed the pros and cons of going somewhere else where she had few friends, but it developed, as it often does in this rather mobile area, that there was no longer any one place where many of her friends were. Most were still alive but scattered all over Southern California. In fact, after talking to realtors and getting some work done on her home, she decided not to leave.

After this point, there were about 10 more sessions spread out over several months as we gradually terminated therapy. Although we both saw considerable room for further improvement in her life situation, there was, in fact, no more change after this point. She had considerable improvement in mood, reduced guilt, increased contact with other people, and increased ability to take care of her personal business. She had largely placed her husband's death in perspective. On the other hand, she had neither positive enjoyment in her life nor much sense of purpose for the remainder of her life.

She still had days in which she felt overwhelmed by depression, although she also had the awareness that these days were episodic and seldom more frequent than one per week. This awareness enabled her to plan her life around these depressed days. She would even joke about them. She had no desire to become active in the local congregation of her church—never attended it, in fact—because she could not picture herself being anything but the pastor. She decided against consulting former mentors in her church about renewed purpose in life. She had no desire to pursue a life review approach in therapy. In summary, she had improved as much as she felt inclined to strive for at this point in her life and was better but not happy.

DISCUSSION

Rapport Building. JoAnn illustrates an interesting set of issues with regard to building rapport in the early sessions of therapy: On the one hand, she was quite familiar with counseling and with psychological ideas. She had studied and read psychology throughout her life and had practiced pastoral counseling herself. In fact, given the beliefs of her church, it would be difficult to distinguish what she called pastoral counseling from many cognitive therapies.

On the other hand, she presented a very different view of her initial problem from the one that I saw. By defining her problem as a need to quit smoking, she was focusing on a specific small behavior, rather than on the more obvious and more psychological problem of adjusting to the loss of her husband. The redefinition of her problem required both education and diplomatic negotiation. First I described what I thought the problem was and why. I then linked my interpretation of the problem to the difficulties that she had with the stop smoking classes.

The diplomacy was expressed in two ways. I continually made it clear that I was describing my view of the situation and that other views could also be correct. I also made it clear that it was up to her to choose what approach she wanted to take in changing her life. With this open negotiation, it took her only a couple of visits to decide to try talking about her husband's death as a way to improve her life. This type of negotiation is common in working with older adults, who frequently do not come into therapy with a psychological explanation for their problems already in mind. Much the same steps were repeated in changing the focus from grieving for a nearly perfect husband to exploring her irritation with his negativity and with some of the decisions that he had made for them before his illness and death.

Techniques in Therapy. Most of the successful work with JoAnn was grief work (cf. Worden, 1982). This largely involved simply encouraging her to recall and talk about her husband, his illness, and the circumstances of the death itself. In JoAnn's case, the blocked emotion was her anger at her husband for the decisions he had made and for the way he handled being ill and dying. Encouraging her to express these feelings helped grief to run its natural course to completion. Acknowledging the deceased as a real human being with faults and good points, as opposed to a perfect spouse, is often part of the cognitive restructuring of grief (Worden, 1982). Idealizing the deceased often indicates some unwillingness to express anger at him or her.

With the emotional issues resolved, the other problem facing her was reconstructing life without him (Rando, 1984; Worden, 1982). Part of this focused on deciding whether to continue to live in Ventura. We pursued a decision-making process, including defining options, exploring options, discussing the decision with others, and beginning to take steps toward moving. At that point, JoAnn decided not to leave, a decision that surprised both of us. Since initial impressions are often based on incomplete consideration of the pros and cons of various options, it often happens that the structured decision-making process leads to an unexpected outcome.

The remainder of the attempted work with JoAnn was in trying to increase the pleasant events in her life, which largely meant increasing contact with friends. While there was some progress in increasing interaction with a few former friends, her decision not to do more in this regard is instructive and not at all unusual among older adults. In this particular instance, it seemed that her need to stay in control and in the role of the helper was more important than the need for closeness.

This need to stay in her accustomed role is perhaps the more curious since she also had no desire to resume being a pastor. She was tired of that professional role and did not have the energy to work on others' problems and look strong while doing it. It seemed to me (and still does) that she could have worked through this dilemma and resolved it in a way that would have enabled her to experience more pleasure; however, it was clearly her decision not to do so.

Gerontological Issues. The primary impact of gerontological expertise in JoAnn's therapy was the recognition of the unfinished grieving as the primary issue confronting her. In general, I do not see this as a major insight or an especially sophisticated one; however, teaching novice therapists and consulting with therapists who have less experience working with the elderly has taught me that many psychotherapists find it easy to miss the importance of a recent death in the client's history. This is particularly pronounced when the client minimizes the importance of the loss, but also occurs when grief is the presenting problem and the therapist finds a different issue to work on.

Although not perhaps an entire issue in itself, the choice of terms used to describe anger when working with older women is consistent enough to deserve some comment. In what is almost certainly a cohort effect, those women who are older now (born before 1920) are usually very reluctant to use the term *anger* to describe their feelings. In general, it is more strategic to simply accept this reluctance and use "softer" terms, like *irritated* or *frustrated*. When these euphemisms seem very weak for a given situation, phrases like "You must have been really, really frustrated" will usually make the point. In general, it is not so much that the existence of the emotional state itself is denied, but that there is considerable discomfort with the use of more aggressive language, especially in women who were well into middle age when the feminist movement of the 1970s made angry women a more generally acceptable notion.

Other gerontological influences are in a sense negative ones and are illustrated by things I did not do with JoAnn that I have seen advocated by therapists who see only the occasional older client. Conventional wisdom in such cases might have dictated encouraging her to move closer to her son or to move into a senior citizens apartment complex or other congregate living. Having an appreciation of the diversity of individual needs and preferences and the wide variety of outcomes of such moves (many resulting in disappointment), I prefer to guide the decision process but not its outcome.

The ending of JoAnn's therapy is instructive for much of both thinking and practice in gerontology. She was clearly isolated geographically and emotionally from former friends, and yet, like many older adults I have known, chose not to work either at making new friends or at reviving old friendships. The naive view that isolation means loneliness, and that friendships are easily made and always worthwhile, is a younger adult worldview that often leads us to prescribe more social interaction for isolated elderly. Karen Rook's work on loneliness (1984) clarifies that loneliness is the combination of isolation and negative affective experience.

In general, older people seem to be able to tolerate time alone better than the young. It seems to me from clinical experience that older adults have a better appreciation of degrees of friendship, the difficulty of finding and making friends, the potential obligations of friendship, and the pain of losing friends and loved ones. In many individual cases, and after many group discussions about making friends, older adults articulate the feeling that it's too difficult to make friends or repair old friendships. The choice to stay alone may not always be understandable to the young (who in some studies report greater subjective loneliness than do the old), but is a viable choice for at least some of the old.

Relationship Issues. JoAnn's relationship to me was generally positive but somewhat complicated by expectations based on her prior professional role. On the one hand, she had some desire to educate and advise me; yet on the other hand, she expected me to criticize her beliefs or minimize her competence as a professional because she had been a minister and I was a secular professional psychologist. As the therapy relationship developed, there was a tendency to ask for direct advice and solutions and to quietly resist the interpretations and directives that were offered. In what I suspect was a general pattern in relating to men, if not to both genders, JoAnn sought out guidance, but then would either ignore it or act in opposition to what was suggested. As suggested by discussions near the end of therapy, this pattern seemed to maintain her sense of control and independence.

On my side, I felt very positively about JoAnn and enjoyed her intelligence, charm, and dry sense of humor. She was sufficiently engaging and her professional background and personal history were so interesting that it was often difficult to stay alert to her resistance. She was highly verbal and skilled at changing the subject with entertaining conversational gambits, so it required considerable vigilance to catch her topic shifts. She was also quite charming and could easily minimize her avoidance of emotional topics and her failure to do homework assignments. Challenging and confronting her felt rather like turning the tables on a well-liked teacher and telling her that she was unprepared for class. It required both concentration and determination to stick to my plans for each session and to make sure that she did as well.

Summary. JoAnn's therapy is an example of a brief therapy that improved her emotional distress considerably, but certainly did not achieve all of my goals for her. It also illustrates a fairly simple use of grief work to overcome depression in a woman who did not originally perceive herself as needing to grieve. The rapport building and relationship aspects of the case show both the need to redefine presenting problems with some older clients and the problems that arise with clients for whom one has high positive regard.

CHAPTER SEVEN

Rena:
Grieving for Children

Rena was in her late 60s when she first came for therapy at our clinic. Although the focus here is on the grief work phase of her therapeutic work, that is not where our contact began. I will begin with some background description of the Senior Outreach team's work with Rena and her two sons.

Our initial contact was with Paul, who came to an adult outpatient clinic in the same mental health center for therapy for depression. Paul had been unhappy about the family's move to California from the Midwest and about the subsequent worsening of his physical condition. Paul had a congenital, progressive physical disorder, which had left his body malformed and which seemed to worsen steadily in its impact on his vision and his ability to walk. He had been more familiar with his surroundings and had more social contacts in the Midwest. His community there had more services for physically disabled persons and more extensive public transportation. Paul was in his 40s and was above-average in intelligence.

Our contact started in two ways: He was assigned to a psychology intern who needed clinical supervision, and it was gradually determined that the only psychologist on staff familiar with physical disability issues was the geropsychologist. Shortly into Paul's therapy the intern felt that intervention was also needed with Paul's mother because of their interdependency, his hostility toward her, and her tendency to overprotect him. The clearest image of this is her walking behind him as they leave the clinic, holding his belt while he walked on canes, with him complaining and cursing constantly.

She was assigned to a clinical social worker in the Outreach program who saw Rena for a year or so, working on her anxiety and stress and her relationship with her son. In these early sessions, Rena was so distressed that she talked rapidly, switched topics frequently, and had trouble concentrating on what the therapist said. Much of the focus was on allowing her to ventilate her feelings and on structuring her speaking and listening, so that she could benefit from therapeutic input and eventually talk constructively with her sons. After a time, she asked for help with her younger son, Bill, who had a similar condition, was in his 30s, and tended to be quiet and withdrawn. The younger son became my client.

In time the intern finished her internship, the social worker took a position in a different clinic, and Rena and Paul became my clients. We continued to work mostly in individual sessions, with occasional conjoint sessions to facilitate communication. They were each so inhibited in expressing emotions in front of the others, and communication was so difficult in conjoint sessions, that individual therapy seemed the most practical approach. The two sons each worked on emotional issues in acceptance of their disability and on ways to take greater control over their lives in a realistic manner.

In Paul's case, this focused mostly on expressing anger and frustration, increasing treatment adherence, and learning a more assertive (less aggressive) style of communicating with his mother. In Bill's case, it involved becoming more open and less passive. For Rena, the work focused on controlling stress, finding ways to have time for herself, and making room for her sons to do more on their own.

As an example of this phase of the work, Paul's walking was becoming worse and he angrily resisted moving from canes to walker and from walker to wheelchair. In the process, he fell often. Rena would rush to his aid, meanwhile explaining why he had fallen. Paul would become infuriated with both the assistance and the explanations of his falls. With work on both sides, she learned to wait while he tried to get up by himself and to reduce her explanations. He learned to remind her to back off, to reduce insults and cursing, and to ask for her help when he knew he needed it.

His move to a wheelchair came after he fell in the shower, during one of Rena's rare 2-hour absences from the home, and lay on the floor until she returned. It is, of course, interesting that he chose to take a shower while she was absent. This also was an important incident in Bill's therapy since he felt guilty about his inability to help. Aside from his own disability, he was thin and frail while Paul was overweight.

A few months later we were working on Paul's anger about progressively failing eyesight. He had also gotten interested in exploring local services and had taken a class at the local community college. One evening a cousin of his, whom I knew personally and professionally, called to inform me that Paul had awakened at night in some distress, gone to the local hospital, and died.

Everyone, myself included, was surprised. Paul had been very disabled, but did not appear to be terminally ill. In fact, his death was never understood any better than the nature of his disorder during life.

Rena's primary emotional reactions at this point were anger and guilt. She was angry with the doctors and the hospital and felt that something more might have been done. She also reviewed repeatedly the time from hearing him call out at night until he got to the hospital; she felt that she might have acted faster, anticipated his distress, or forced the paramedics to arrive faster. She felt some sorrow at his death and regret that their relationship had never become more calm.

As is common in late-life grief, grieving for Paul brought out unresolved grief from earlier stages of her life. She began to bring out memories of her deceased husband, who had died some 15 years previously. He had been dominant, aggressive, and distant. She apparently had dealt with his death by focusing attention on her sons, with no time left to experience feelings about losing him. Paul had moved into a similar role with her. The relationships had become sufficiently alike that it was not always immediately clear whom she was missing or grieving for. Paul's absence did allow for her to develop more of a relationship with Bill.

A few months after Paul's death, Rena was diagnosed with a cancer of the throat. This provoked tremendous anxiety and a reluctance to either confront the problem or have the surgery. It developed that Rena had an unexpressed (possibly even unconscious) conviction that, in exchange for caring for her sons, she herself was immune to illness. Up to this point, she had been nearly totally free from common illnesses like colds and the chronic illnesses of late life. Now she had to confront her own illness and the possibility of death.

She came through the surgery well, but was left with some difficulty swallowing and speaking. She was an extremely resistive patient with her rehabilitation therapists, being impatient that she was not immediately better and becoming hostile about doing assignments. In general, the tone was, "I'm over 70, why should I need to learn to swallow?" She was encouraged to express anger with me rather than with the oncologist and the speech therapist, to comply with assignments, and to discuss the realities of her situation.

She also gradually made the connection between her reaction to her rehabilitation and the way her sons had responded to theirs. Unfortunately, this belated realization also produced guilt that she had not more fully realized this while Paul was alive. I was also involved in her guilt in that she often expressed that I had tried to get her to see her sons' point of view. I was personally uncomfortable at the delayed effect of an interpretation that would have helped at one time, but made her feel worse at this time.

During this same period of time, Bill was working on issues related to his brother's death and his mother's illness and possible death. It had never occurred to him that his mother could be ill or die. Both possibilities caused considerable anxiety and also a need to change his own identity in their relationship. It was, in short, his job to be ill and hers to be the caregiver, and the idea that the job could change was novel and changed his self-concept. Once past the initial anxiety, he welcomed the chance to do some things for her and to coach her on ways to handle disability and rehabilitation.

Bill responded to his older brother's death by becoming convinced that he too would die soon. He believed, without objective evidence, that he was progressing faster than Paul had. (If anything, he seemed healthier.) His mother's illness brought up considerable anxiety in that it had never occurred to him that he might outlive her, and the thought of living in a skilled nursing facility was horrifying to him. He also grieved for his older brother

who had been a role model for him and with whom he had identified. We worked on differentiating himself from Paul, on examining possible alternatives for himself if he did outlive his mother,
and on his own possible death. In Bill's case, however, the greater
anxiety was in the possibility that he might go on living, rather
than that he would die soon.

Rena gradually came to accept Paul's death, along with some
resolution of feelings about her deceased husband. She completed
rehabilitation and began to socialize again. She and Bill were relating fairly well, and therapy was beginning to wrap up.

After a family holiday dinner with her brother and various
cousins, Bill began to choke. Paramedics were called. He was
taken to the hospital and died.

Grief was renewed; Rena missed both of her sons and was faced
with an empty house for the first time in her life. Her grief for Bill
was mostly expressed in dreams and in a strong sense of his presence in the house, which continued for months afterward. In therapy, the most salient and most difficult part of the work was her
search for a new identity. In this search, life review played a significant role.

Rena had grown up in a Jewish ghetto in a large midwestern
city, the child of Russian-Jewish immigrants. The men were central in the family, and she was taught to serve both her father and
her brother. Grandparents joined the family in her early teen
years, and she felt nearly invisible after that because her mother's
attention focused on caring for the elderly parents and she became an assistant. Oddly, given her impressions of her family of
origin, she went to college and got a social service degree.

She married a merchant and established a home of her own. She
had a son who was completely healthy. At the time I saw her, he
was a successful professional man in the Midwest. A few years
later (when Rena was 24) Paul was born and she became devoted
to learning about his problems, seeking diagnoses, and seeking
the best possible care. Several years later, the family doctor ad-
vised that "lightning couldn't strike twice" and she had a third
child in an attempt to take some of her attention from Paul. The
third child was Bill. As part of this review, she was able to become

extremely angry at this physician, albeit 45 years later and 2,000 miles away. She had several dreams and daytime visual fantasies of attacking and dismembering this man.

While raising her children, she was able to find good services for them, including special classes and camps. After high school, Paul held a job for a while. Out of these experiences, she returned to school and got a master's degree and worked in special education for several years. After retirement, she decided to come to California to be closer to family. She had, in short, devoted her life, from age 24 to age 70, to the care of her two disabled sons. She had never expected to outlive them and had no plans for life as Rena alone.

During this time and as a result of conversations in therapy, she reestablished contact with some former friends by letter, telephone, and visit. These contacts helped her to establish other images of herself, as a competent teacher, professional person, and friend. She became more involved in the Temple, especially in related organizations and in religious symbols for memorializing her sons. Some unfinished business with her sons was handled by visits to their graves, where she talked with them about how she handled caring for them. For several months she continued these visits as a way of remembering.

Attempts to seek new friends or to integrate herself into discussion groups in senior centers or into a therapy group were all unsuccessful. She decided that the costs of new friendship were too high, even though she continued to feel considerable loneliness. Most interactions with other older women would lead to the subject of grandchildren, and her major regret about her life was the absence of grandchildren. Bill and Paul had never been able to have children. Her healthy son, married to a busy professional woman, had chosen not to have children.

Over a period of several months, she chose social and volunteer activities with which she was comfortable. She gradually terminated therapy. She is an active and relatively healthy older woman who is still lonely and still very unhappy about the absence of grandchildren in her life.

DISCUSSION

Rapport Building. Rena represents an atypical instance in that my therapy with her began as a result of a transfer from another therapist. In many ways this meant that she was already "broken in" to the work of therapy. In fact, my ability to work with her was, I believe, dependent upon this earlier therapy. Her first therapist was a clinical social worker, who displayed enormous patience with highly anxious and difficult clients and worked very effectively with them. Rena had become considerably less anxious, her speech had slowed a great deal, and she was able to listen and absorb my input to a much greater extent after working with the other therapist. Even with these changes, when Rena first came in for help, she had an interpersonal style that I found very difficult to tolerate, much less work with.

On the other hand, we had several issues to deal with in the early part of our therapy. She had lost a therapist whom she felt very close to and comfortable with. I was very different from the other therapist in gender, appearance, personality, and therapeutic orientation. We had to explore all of these differences in addition to her feelings about the first therapist's leaving to take another job. Over the course of three or four sessions, she decided that she could work with me and make the best out of the differences I would bring to working on her problems. For several weeks, we would continue to consider "what M_____ would have said about this" as well as my input.

It was also important to delineate my role with her and each of her sons as well as working with them altogether at times. While it is clearly better theoretically to have more than one therapist involved in working with family members in this way, the fact was that we were severely understaffed for a couple of years, and there was no one available to join with me in conjoint work with this family. I suspect such external contingencies frequently arise and dictate therapeutic strategy. We clarified the nature and limits of confidentiality in this situation. My basic working premise is that I do not discuss each person's individual progress or process with the others, but I also do not guarantee confidentiality of content or of a specific problem unless it is specifically negotiated. When one is working with a couple or a family system, broad promises of confidentiality for each individual severely handicap the work of promoting open communication within the system.

We also discussed the probability that she and her sons might feel jealous of me and perceive favoritism on my part. I also invited everyone to call me on any perceived tendency on my part to take sides with any one of them consistently. This invitation included a warning that if I was being fair, each of them would feel I was on someone else's side part of the time. Fortunately, each of them was sufficiently socialized to therapy by this time that these rules and warnings were quickly understood and used.

Techniques in Therapy. The work with Rena and her sons, while they lived, largely consisted of intertwined individual and family sessions that were designed to improve communication and more equally distribute power in the family. These interventions were also guided by a rehabilitation model in that our goal was to maximize everyone's independence by matching daily functioning to actual ability. In some instances this meant encouraging her sons to do more and Rena to let them. At other times, it meant encouraging acceptance of disability, such as Paul's acceptance of the wheelchair.

The death of each son clearly occasioned a need for grief work. The grieving for Paul also occasioned a realignment of the family system, with a new role for Bill. Grieving for Bill necessitated a redefinition of Rena's identity, which had been as the mother and caregiver for more than 40 years. The fact of the sons' disabilities had eliminated adolescent rebellion and young adult separation from the family. Rena had never experienced the leaving-the-nest stage of family development nor the empty-nest marriage (Carter & McGoldrick, 1988). Rather than losing her sons to independence and their own families, she lost two of them to death and found herself alone and with few concrete plans for her life.

Rena's bout with cancer and rehabilitation demonstrates the psychological reality of Rando's (1984) separation of grieving from preparing for one's own death. Rena was much better prepared for grieving than for facing illness and death herself. It came as a complete surprise to her that she could become ill, need hospitalization and rehabilitation, and might die of cancer. Her focus on caring for her sons and their extreme disability had shielded her from attending to the changes in her own body over the years, which stimulate others to contemplate the finitude of their lives.

She also had implicitly taken her good health as sign of a bargain that she would be immune to illness and death in exchange for caring for her sons. There was considerable denial, anger, and depression to work through as she learned to accept this insult to her physical integrity and think constructively about what she wanted from her remaining years.

Gerontological Issues. Rena's family poses some intriguing challenges to our typical conceptions of older people and older families in gerontology. First and foremost, here is an example of an often-neglected phenomenon: an older woman caring for her disabled children, rather than the presumably more typical picture of the frail elder being dependent upon younger generations. Secondary to that fact is all of its implications for the life cycle of the family and for Rena's personal development for her adult years. The family system with mother caring for dependent children did not change for her, as it more often does with children maturing and leaving home. She never experienced that separation and the consequent individuation for herself. She never experienced the empty-nest marriage with her husband. She delayed grieving for him for nearly 20 years after his death. She never became a grandmother.

A family systems perspective, often lacking in gerontology, is helpful in understanding Paul's critical and angry style with his mother as being due in part to his taking over his father's role, and Rena's being comfortable with having a critical male figure in her life (Brown, 1988; Hall, 1981). It was also very helpful in understanding and guiding the changes in roles and relationships following Paul's death.

Some degree of gerontological sophistication is implicit in understanding the value of her continuing to live alone and in California, close to her brother and his family, rather than encouraging her to move close to her son. Sibling relationships can be just as important, and often more supportive, than relationships with children in later life.

Our search for meaningful activities to replace the full-time work of caregiving was guided by an understanding of her unique interests across her life span. Thus we focused on exploring volunteer work with children and teens, renewing religious interests, enjoying opportunities to travel, and so on. Rena had never socialized with or identified with older adults to any degree and found the common focus on discussing grandchildren painful, so encouraging her to pursue aging network activities would have been unhelpful. She also clearly preferred more intense personal involvement to larger-scale social or recreational activities.

Relationship Issues. The most salient issues for me in therapy with Rena revolved around my own reactions to the death of her sons, who were also my clients. Paul's death surprised me, saddened me, and annoyed me. The annoyance came from the interruption of our therapy work together and the fact that therapy was very clearly unfinished. In fact, we had been rather stuck for the couple of months prior to his death. I had wanted to accomplish more with him and for him, and his sudden demise left me feeling cheated and unfinished. It required considerable care on my part to distinguish my feelings and my grief from Rena's when we worked together on completing her grief for Paul.

She also was surprised and felt unfinished with him. Her emotions were based on different reasons and a much longer and closer relationship. I would at times find myself wanting to share my feelings, assuming that we missed the same things or saw him in the same way, when a second thought suggested that it was more appropriate to encourage her to express her own feelings more fully or explore and explain more completely what she missed about Paul. While at times it was helpful to acknowledge that I was missing him or had felt shocked by his death, or to share mutual memories, for the most part it seemed far more helpful to make it clear that it was her grief that the sessions focused on, not mine.

In contrast, Bill's death was a surprise to me, but I did feel finished with his therapy and rather pleased with what we had accomplished together. There was also a curious sense of rightness to his death in that he had clearly expected it and desired it. I had been convinced that he was wrong in predicting that he would die in the near future, but could understand why he felt more comfortable with death than with outliving his mother. Rena was in this instance much more distressed and upset than was I. Again, it was necessary to follow her emotions and thoughts, rather than imposing my own on her.

One of the things that psychotherapy with older adults has taught me is that death is essentially unpredictable. When I started working with the elderly, I expected that many clients would die, but I have experienced fewer such deaths than I anticipated. I have learned that people who look very frail and very close to death can live for years, and this is perhaps the saddest knowledge that I have acquired in this career. I have also been confronted with the sudden death of clients whom I thought of as being among the healthiest and most active of my clients. Each death has its own emotional impact on me as the therapist.

I have been fortunate throughout my career to have worked within the context of a team that acted like a team. The members of that team were people who could listen to my concerns, as well as people who would make me talk when I needed to and did not want to. I have done the same for others and have observed that some people are unable to have several clients die and continue to engage in therapeutic relationships with older clients who are perceived as likely to die. The general lack of attention to this issue in working with the elderly is disturbing and tragic.

Summary. Rena's life and therapy remind us of overlooked issues in working with the older family: the older person as caregiver for dependent adult children and the older person's grief for the death of children. The work with disability and with grief in a family context shows the variety of meanings that death can have, even within one family grieving for the same person. The experience of the death of clients is painful. Both training and appropriately supportive teamwork are important in assisting the therapist who confronts such pain.

CHAPTER EIGHT

Rose:
Coping With Delayed Grief

Rose was in her mid-50s when we met. She lived alone and was retired on disability from a job as a bus driver. Her completely white hair and somewhat vaguely defined disabilities gave the impression of a much older woman. She identified herself as a "senior" and generally associated with people 15 and more years older than herself. Not infrequently, one of these chronologically older friends would be challenged as not being old enough to qualify for senior rates on transportation or for meals; Rose, who actually was too young to qualify, was never challenged.

I knew Rose for several months as a member of a therapy group that I co-led during my internship years in clinical psychology. We began individual sessions at the suggestion of the other therapist in the group, who felt that Rose needed more individual attention to cope with depression and limited social activity after the death of her main social companion for activities, a woman close to her own age.

She minimized the impact of the loss of her friend, whom she characterized as scarcely more than an acquaintance. She acknowledged feeling depressed, but was very reluctant to see any connection between daily events and changes in her mood. She seemed to prefer to see her depression as an unexplainable occurrence in her life. She was subject to marked mood variations, all at a level that could be characterized as varying between depressed and very depressed. She gradually completed assignments on monitoring her daily moods and admitted that I saw patterns to her moods that went with various events in her life. Attempts to go further and identify pleasurable events ran aground on her insistence that nothing was enjoyable for her.

Shifting to what had been pleasurable in the past, she very quickly stated that she mostly had enjoyed working. We discussed the chances of her returning to work, which she felt were good, although she did state that her doctor was opposed to it. There was also the problem that part-time work was not an option, since her disability checks would be discontinued if she were considered able to work. She also expressed pessimism about anyone hiring her with her record, since previous attempts to return to work had not gone well. She was also seeing a psychiatrist at the same clinic for antidepressant medication. He warned me before our next visit that prior attempts to return to work had in fact resulted in Rose's being admitted to the hospital (for medical reasons).

She acknowledged this pattern and reviewed it with me when I brought it up, although she expressed little concern over it. At this point she acknowledged only that her doctor saw her as having high blood pressure and a rapid heartbeat. She characterized her problems in returning to work as becoming exhausted. I thought it wiser to seek other pleasurable events, and we identified a few social activities at church and volunteer work that she could do at church. Although she reported extreme effort to do these things, and frequent failures, her mood improved to the point that she seemed to vary between mild depression and more severe depressions.

Rose's more severe depressions were accompanied by frequent suicidal thoughts and, in fact, she was rarely free of suicidal thoughts for a full day. She had no history of attempts, even though she reported serious suicidal ideation for years previously.

I became aware of her migraine headaches only because she came in for a session with one. She described having had extensive treatments, but said that nothing had worked. We began relaxation training, with very little reported effect.

At about this time in her therapy, after approximately 6 months of individual sessions, I considered termination because I felt that we had accomplished little and I had few ideas about what might be accomplished. When I brought this up with Rose, I was surprised to discover that she felt the sessions had been helpful, although she was hard put to say how. Her comments, about the slowness of her progress and her own stubbornness about doing things that I suggested, displayed a wry sense of humor.

Several things influenced my decision to continue with Rose in therapy. On a conceptual level, I had begun to realize that Rose was dealing with chronic problems of isolation, poor health, and disability. While I had been trained in behaviorally oriented therapy to consider lack of progress after a few months an indication that therapy was not working and should be terminated, I had also been taught that environmental contingencies controlled behavior, and I saw little change in the set of circumstances that controlled Rose's behavior. My clinical supervisor at that time also called my attention to the likelihood that direct behavioral prescription motivated resistance by engaging her stubbornness and suggested that I might work around it with less direct methods and engage her sense of humor as a positive asset. Although each session was slow and difficult going, I also found that I liked Rose as a person and was intrigued by her perception of slow and worthwhile progress.

We went on for several months in this vein with continued slow progress. An unexpected visit from one of her sons brought a sharp increase in depressed mood at a time when she was otherwise doing quite well—which is to say that mood variations were from flat to moderately depressed, and she had occasional days without suicidal thoughts. Exploration of this change in mood led to her admitting, after several sessions, that while she resented her children's neglecting her, their visits often made her depressed.

As she described specific examples, it became clear to me, but not to her, that her children often made her angry. I tried to work for clear communication of what she wanted from them and for more expression of feeling in sessions about them, but with no progress. I did learn more about her history as it was intertwined with relating to her children. She gradually acknowledged some "irritation" with them at times. She would smile acknowledgement when I would amend this to say, "You sound like you were *extremely* irritated that time," but refused any attempt to engage her in more direct expression of feelings.

What emerged as history included the following: All of her children were, in her opinion, having problems. One son, who lived within 100 miles, was overweight, overworked, and unhealthy. Another son had severe pain from arthritis and had relocated and changed careers with little success. Her daughter was unhappily married, obese, and often taking medication that was prescribed, but which Rose thought was unnecessary. She disapproved of the way they raised their children, while simultaneously expressing extreme guilt about the way she had raised them.

With regard to this last, she related that during their childhood she had been strict with them. She had often been ill and bedbound; but when she was healthy, she had worked very hard outside the home. She worried that she had been both overly strict and remote and unavailable. There had been little expression of emotion in the family. Her first husband had died after a year-long bout with cancer when the children were finishing high school. One of the children had been "kicked out" of the house by her husband not long before his illness, and they had not reconciled before he died. As he went to the hospital for the last time, he made her promise not to grieve for him. She had done her best to keep this promise.

She remarried a few years later, with all the children expressing relief that she had someone to be with who could take care of her. She felt that they had remained distant ever since, even though she had been divorced for several years and her second husband had remarried.

Therapy at this point was extremely slow. She was more depressed than she had been in several months and more resistant to talking about these issues than she had been about anything since the early days of the therapy. At one point she arrived for a visit extremely confused and babbling in a disoriented way. An emergency consultation with the clinic psychiatrist established that she had started a new medication for which this was a not uncommon side-effect. I drove her home and saw that her mobile home, which she always described as a disgraceful mess, was actually quite tidy, clean, and well organized. She continued after this, as she had before, to resist giving permission for us to communicate directly with her primary care physician.

Around this time, I had become fascinated with visualization techniques and the strategy of using visual imagery with clients who were resistant to discussing emotionally laden topics verbally (Erickson, 1980; Singer, 1974). Using a mild trance-induction and the instruction to visualize a blank movie screen and simply allow images to appear, I explored for times when she had been happy, relaxed, and confident. She described a fireside scene in several of these sessions and gradually revealed, with tears in her eyes, that this had been a very happy time with Hugh, her first husband. Thus I realized that she was still grieving for Hugh, who had been dead for more than 15 years at this point.

Using both the visual blank screen technique and verbal guided recollection, we proceeded over the next few months to discuss both her relationship with Hugh and his death. He had been a good provider and very supportive of her through various illnesses and in her struggles to work. He had been rather authoritarian with the children, and she had sometimes supported them behind his back or intervened more directly on their behalf. He had been diagnosed with cancer at a time when he seemed quite healthy, and had died suddenly after a few months of illness. They had rarely been overtly emotional or affectionate, and he had insisted throughout his illness that they not discuss it and that she would not cry about it. On his last night, he literally made her promise not to grieve for him. Having never been very expressive herself, she found it natural to follow these directives.

After 2 years of therapy with very little overt emotional expression, Rose would glow as she talked about good times with Hugh, and tears would well up in her eyes and she would choke up and become silent while talking about his death. She refused my attempts to have her attend a grieving group because she was unwilling to show so much feeling in front of others. In contrast to her feelings about Hugh, her second husband seemed to arouse no feelings whatsoever. She seemed neither to have felt strongly about him nor to have a sense of loss about the divorce. My impression was that her relationship with Hugh was so strong that her arrangement with Hank was more instrumental than affectionate.

As her grief work drew to a close, I began to explore her recollections of illness. It developed that Rose had developed polio when quite young and had spent months in a children's hospital at about the age of 9. Her parents were fairly unsophisticated, hard-working people. Her father was a foreman on Southern California citrus ranches. Although the doctors had predicted a life of disability and chronic pain, she had determined to return to a normal life and school. While she did have frequent absences from school and bouts of pain, she returned to normal walking and a relatively normal life that became one of overachieving. She recalled herself as a workaholic at all of her jobs, demanding that she do all work that needed to be done and not being content to do just her own job.

It was this style that often led to physical incapacitation and repeated hospital admissions. She had perfected the stoic attitude, which was her family heritage, and resisted expressing pain, depression, or any emotion. She had also overlearned the habit of covering for her disability. At the time I knew her she had been in pain for five decades.

After reviewing this aspect of her history, I began to work more consistently with her on letting go of the idea of returning to work. Although she was often irritated with me during these sessions, after repeated confrontation with the facts of her own life history, she gradually acknowledged that she could not work without putting herself in the hospital. This realization was followed by more realistic planning about how she wanted to spend her life from this point on. She chose a variety of church and community volunteer activities, explicitly rejecting more socially oriented activities or the idea of dating again. Some time later she did get more involved with her second husband after his current wife died.

At this point, some 5 years into our therapeutic relationship, Rose no longer seemed depressed to me, although she often had periods of severe fatigue when she would be housebound, if not bedbound. Her physician of several years found these episodes unremarkable, and Rose herself was inclined to see them as related to her depression or due to stress. I was concerned because the fatigue had seemed to continue and grow worse while the rest of her depressive symptoms had lessened: She was very infrequently troubled by suicidal thoughts; depressive thinking had nearly vanished; appetite and sleep were normal for her; and while seldom happy, she no longer felt sad.

After a consultation within our own clinic with a geriatric nurse practitioner and further discussion about her physician, whom she had often criticized as inattentive over the years but had never considered leaving, Rose asked for a referral and was seen by a young family practice physician who had consulted with members of our team during her residency. Diagnosed as having a heart condition, Rose was referred to a cardiologist and soon had surgery and follow-up medical treatment for her problem. Her energy level improved rather markedly after this. I have no way of knowing how long this medical problem had existed or what its contribution was to symptoms we had both interpreted as depression.

After a few months of reducing the frequency of our visits and discussing our long, affectionate therapy relationship, we terminated therapy visits. Not long after this termination, we resumed therapy because her older sister was near death, and Rose was visiting her frequently. Her sister did, in fact, die within a few months, and we discussed this relationship and its impact on her life. Rose had long looked up to and been somewhat dominated by her sister. She could not believe that her "stronger sister" had died before she had. She also felt that she was at the greatest risk of dying now that her sister was gone.

Rose also began to receive notes from her son in Washington State. He was in therapy for a severe depression and had developed the conviction that he had been abused as a child and wanted Rose to tell him about it. He had no memories of the presumed incident. She had no idea what he was talking about, but we reviewed her recollections of child-raising and her general sense of guilt about her children, and discussed ways to prepare for a coming visit to both children in Washington State, who lived within about 20 miles of one another, but never visited and seldom spoke on the phone. The trip did not go especially well since her son was very angry and confrontive without being able to say anything very specific.

Not long after this visit, her daughter, who was about 40 years old, died. Rose was shocked, grief-stricken, and (for once) openly angry at her daughter's HMO physician, whom Rose characterized as willing to give her daughter any medication to keep her quiet. She further thought that the doctor had long ago decided that her daughter was a hypochondriac and had ignored warning symptoms of heart trouble. In fact, when she got the autopsy report, her daughter had died of a progressively developing heart disorder, which is commonly recognized early on. Rose encouraged her son-in-law to file a lawsuit, which he did.

We worked through her grief over the loss of her daughter and her guilt about her failures as a mother. This time her guilt was focused on the physical condition of her children, all of whom had serious chronic physical conditions and were prone to avoid taking care of themselves. In fact, they tended to engage in high-risk behaviors, such as overeating, overworking, medication abuse, and noncompliance with medical treatment when they did seek it.

Her guilt over their actual illnesses was irrational and relatively easy to deal with in therapy. Their manner of handling their conditions was so clearly similar to hers that guilt could be attenuated only by pointing out that she had learned her behavior from her parents, and having her do some "make up work." She talked with her surviving children about what she had learned about coping with chronic illness and what they should learn from their sister's death. Not too surprisingly, her death had motivated the whole family, and there were some changes in her sons' health behaviors.

At this point, it seemed to me that she was ready for termination from therapy. She, however, was very reluctant to leave, so we compromised on her moving to group therapy. She attended regularly and was a good supportive group member. At times she brought up family-related issues on her own. She was still attending group when I resigned from the clinic to work at USC.

DISCUSSION

Rapport Building. Rose was both easy and difficult in terms of establishing rapport in therapy. She had considerable experience with both individual and group therapy and certainly knew how to play the role of client. She was, in general, passively agreeable in sessions, with little compliance in between sessions during the early phase of therapy. In another sense, I feel that the relationship only began developing several months into therapy, when I discussed termination with her the first time. In retrospect, it seems that trust developed very gradually and that each step of therapy and each decision to open up more about her life came slowly and only after the testing represented in the work up to that point. That is, she began to discuss her children only after we had made some definite, slow progress in ameliorating her depression. We worked on her grief for her first husband only after having worked on other family relationships.

Techniques in Therapy. Rose's therapy lasted several years and is perhaps most notable for having embraced a variety of therapeutic strategies and techniques, as we moved through different phases of resolving her depression. The first phase was a very cognitive-behavioral approach, with a particular emphasis on modifying her depressive thinking patterns and finding appropriate outside activities by considering what she enjoyed doing now and what she had considered pleasurable in the past.

This application of pleasant events theory was modified somewhat by rehabilitation perspectives, in that Rose's history clearly ruled out the activity she considered most pleasurable: working. After deciding that was not an option, the question moved to "What is the next most pleasurable thing you could do?" That part of the therapy also highlights an important perspective from behavioral therapy approaches: Rose could not be as happy as she might have liked, so she was inclined to give up; however, my perspective was that she could be considerably happier than she was at the beginning of therapy. In working with the elderly, it is essential to remember that life can virtually always be improved, even when past activities and levels of satisfaction are, in fact, no longer attainable.

The next phase of the therapy was based on family systems perspectives and communications skills training (Carter & McGoldrick, 1988; Gottman, Notarius, Gonzo, & Markman, 1976). We discussed her family network and its history and looked for ways to improve her communication with her children. Her anger and guilt had to be acknowledged and expressed to me before she could start to express herself more clearly to her children. She gradually was able to both ask for assistance and also decline offers of help that she did not want. She became more sympathetic to her children as she began to perceive some of their communication problems as similar to her own. For example, no one in the family was comfortable talking about emotions, so all emotional discussions were awkward and characterized by rough attempts at being humorous. She also came to acknowledge that she disapproved of them in many ways and had to choose between the disapproval and the desire to be close to them.

The use of relaxation methods and visual imagery proved very helpful in circumventing her fairly sophisticated verbal defensive strategies. She simply would not talk about feelings, but could visualize them and visualize emotionally laden scenes. This proved helpful in initiating and completing her grieving for her first husband. For her, grief work meant expressing considerable sadness and finally anger that Hugh had left her. She also had to excuse herself for not living up to the promise to him that she would not grieve. This work with Rose convinced me that unresolved grief has no time limit, nor does the intensity of the feeling diminish with time. Unfinished grief stays unfinished. Rose scarcely finished grieving for Hugh when she was confronted with the loss of her sister, and then her daughter, in quick succession. For Rose, grief work was primarily emotional, and the reconstructive phase of grieving was mostly focused on improved relationships with her children to the extent possible. She also came to see, through our family systems analysis of his death, that it meant something very different to her children. They had lost a father in the midst of the battles they were fighting with him as teenagers and young adults; she was the one who had lost a supportive husband. His death and their inability to grieve together had driven them apart in ways that were difficult to overcome, even 15 years later (Brown, 1988).

The contribution of physical illness to her apparent depression is important to note. She had an unrecognized illness, which certainly accounted for some of her fatigue and depressed mood. Her symptoms were more recognizable after the depression had lifted somewhat. She was also much more amenable to seeking better medical care and complying with treatment when her depression had lifted. She had been dissatisfied with her physician for years, but, being depressed, had felt that it did not matter whether she did anything about it. While in principle it is always preferable to have physical illness diagnosed before treating psychological problems, in work with older adults, physical symptoms are not infrequently hidden by depressed mood or by the client's refusal to seek medical help, which, in turn, may be rooted in depression.

Gerontological Issues. Perhaps the essential gerontological issue that Rose illustrates is the nature of the social perception of age. Much of the time that I knew her, Rose was less than 60 years old. In spite of this, she perceived herself, and was readily seen by others, as "old." One incident she related often is that, while having lunch with a friend who was more than 70, they asked for the senior citizen discount; her friend was asked for proof of age and Rose was not.

Rose is probably best understood as a person who suffered from chronic illness and chronic pain her entire life. Yet she can readily be seen as someone who is "old for her age." Her willingness to not only accept this designation but also exaggerate it is intriguing. For example, Rose tinted her hair to make it more white, rather than coloring it for a more youthful appearance. In her instance, much of this identification with age had to do with wanting to avoid further romantic entanglements in her life.

Rose also clearly illustrates the multiplicity of problems that is more characteristic of later life. During her counseling, we worked on rehabilitation and illness issues; grieving for her husband, sister, and daughter; and a complex of later-life family issues. We also took an active role in referring her for medical diagnosis and treatment. In some areas the outcome of counseling was positive change in her life: improved communication with her children, a greater range of emotional expression, less experienced pain (including the disappearance of migraines). In other areas, the emphasis was acceptance of limitation, especially giving up on working as a viable option. Given her personal history, even this acceptance might equally be seen as giving up a self-destructive pattern of overwork and rehospitalization. Her problems were also chronic rather than acute in nature. While the problems of younger adults are often acute crises, the stressors of later life are often longer lasting chronic problems, which produce chronic distress and require different coping responses (Felton & Revenson, 1987; Pearlin, Turner, & Semple, 1989; Pearlin, Mullan, Semple, & Skaff, 1990).

Rose's grief for her first husband points to the importance of grief and unresolved grief in the lives of those who have had loved ones die. In my experience, new therapists and therapists unfamiliar with gerontology and with grief work often overlook the importance of a history that includes a loved one dying near the time of onset of depressive symptoms. This tendency is more pronounced when the death occurred several years ago, even when the symptoms have been relatively constant for those several years. Unresolved grief can last for decades and is an example of Freud's dictum about the timeless nature of the unconscious. This failure to perceive death as an important life event may be one of the most basic consequences of either the therapist's discomfort with death-related issues or the therapist's lack of life experience with the loss of loved ones.

Relationship Issues. The length of my relationship with Rose is the most salient aspect of that relationship for me. Having been trained to do brief therapy, and still tending to be ideologically committed to the concept that briefer therapy is better, it is curious to me that I saw Rose nearly continuously for more than 10 years. I liked her, respected her viewpoint on many issues, enjoyed her sense of history with me, and shared her sense of humor.

With all of this positive feeling going for us, I wonder to what extent the length of therapy was a function of her very real and very long-standing problems with depression, chronic pain, and chronic illness, compounded by the multiple deaths in her immediate family. It is likely that it was due in part to the fact that we enjoyed talking to one another and could not or would not come to terms with the idea that the therapy was completed and should come to an end. I never liked to think of terminating therapy with her, missed her when we did terminate, and was glad to see her again when she returned. I cannot, however, think of anyone in my personal life whom she either reminds me of or substituted for. At my initiation, we did, in fact, discuss termination of therapy and also transfer to another therapist on several occasions. It is still unclear to me whether therapy lasted so long because her problems continued or because of the positive countertransference.

I think that at times during the grief work for Hugh, Rose related to me as her first husband at an earlier age. Later I feel that there were times when she identified me as a somewhat more positive version of her older son. These mild transferential reactions tended to facilitate the therapy and resolved naturally.

Summary. Rose represents an example of someone making significant changes slowly over a long period of time. She had a long and difficult life, but was able to make positive change in therapy. Those changes made her more active socially and as a volunteer, improved her family relationships, and enabled her to seek medical attention.

CHAPTER NINE

Fred:
Sexual Counseling With Older Men

Fred was in his early 60s when he was referred to me, by another psychologist in the same department, for help with sexual counseling. A former teacher, Fred had been retired on disability for many years because of manic-depressive illness. He had been stable on lithium and had occasional visits with the psychologist to discuss relationship issues and stress management. He had not been hospitalized nor had a manic episode in more than 10 years when I met him. A bright, articulate, easy-going man, he lived with his elderly mother and an aunt in the family home in a small city and drove a senior center transportation van a few hours each week.

His specific problem for our sessions was partial erectile dysfunction. He was sexually active with a younger girlfriend (forty-something) and very much enjoyed giving her pleasure. He was frustrated with his inability to achieve a full erection and reported that his girlfriend felt bad that they did not have intercourse and that he did not have orgasms. He perceived this feeling on her part not as pressure to do more, but rather as a feeling that he did so much to satisfy her that she wanted to return the favor. He described their relationship as stable and otherwise satisfactory to both of them. They had a set pattern of times when they could visit, since both had other obligations with family and work, and neither felt pressure to make the relationship more formal.

I verified that he had discussed his problem with his physician and with the prescribing psychiatrist, and that neither felt there was a physical cause or that his medication would account for the problem. He also reported occasional nocturnal and morning erections, which were not associated with erotic feelings. I described the nature of the counseling and my feeling that it was essential that his girlfriend come in as well. He said he would discuss it with her. He felt she would be willing, but they kept their relationship secret for professional reasons. I discussed confidentiality with him, but also pointed out that even though we would be meeting in a different city, it was a public building and we could not be certain who they would see in the halls or the waiting room.

We discussed his sexual history. He had no unusual experiences or problems learning about sex or with sexual activity as a young man. He had been married once, and sex was neither very good nor very bad. There had been periods of sexual inactivity in his life. He had stopped sexual activity for several years after his hospitalization for mania. His first attempt at sex after this lull had been initiated by a female friend to whom he was not greatly attracted. After a pleasant evening together, she had rather suddenly, as he experienced it, proposed that they sleep together and was more insistent and aggressive than he had previously experienced with a woman. When he was obviously unaroused, she had been vocal about her disappointment and made some disparaging remarks about his manhood.

Since that time, his few encounters had resulted in weak arousal and partial erections. He continued to enjoy giving pleasure to women he was attracted to, and reported generally good reviews on his skills at giving orgasms with manual and oral stimulation. Until his current girlfriend, he had not met a woman who would continue the relationship without intercourse. In spite of this (in my view) fairly clear-cut history, he was reluctant to see the problem as caused by performance anxiety, beginning with the one difficult experience.

A few weeks later, Fred came in with his girlfriend. Her account of their relationship and their sexual life was essentially identical to his, which was a good sign for the success of the counseling. She was a professional woman, separated from her husband who travelled a lot and who was having an acknowledged affair with a woman in another city. For several reasons, she and her husband were not ready to either divorce or publicly acknowledge the separation. In the meantime, she felt her relationship with Fred was ideal in intensity and time commitment. She seemed concerned about being able to give him pleasure without being pressuring about his performance. They were able to discuss their sexual life openly with one another and with me in a candid and nondefensive manner.

Following a modified Masters and Johnson (1970) approach to sexual counseling, I told them to forget about having intercourse for the next several weeks. I also told them to focus as little as possible on his physical arousal or lack of same and instead to concentrate on having fun. In some detail I explained that trying to have better sex is like trying to go to sleep or forcing yourself to relax: It simply doesn't work. They both accepted the rules and the concept quite readily. I directed them to concentrate for the next 2 weeks on nongenital pleasure for him: backrubs, searching for other erogenous zones, and so on.

On the next visit, they expressed satisfaction with the change in their activities. He felt much more relaxed when they were together, and she was enjoying learning more about his body. They were able to engage in playfully redefining pleasure for him in both of their minds. They had also noticed some increase in the size of his penis during sex play.

We continued this pattern for another 2 weeks and then moved to non-goal-oriented genital play. In other words, without planning to achieve an erection and with intercourse still "forbidden," she was allowed to stimulate his genitals directly. On their next several visits, they reported increasing enjoyment of this activity and a gradual acceptance on her part that he really meant it when he said he enjoyed this without the release of orgasm. Women relating to older men often have considerable relearning to do: A lifetime of experience with men having orgasms virtually all the time, and early adulthood learning (from male partners) that arousal without release is painful or extremely distressing, must be unlearned in order to accept older men, who may not always climax and who do not have the same degree of felt urgency about orgasm.

As they continued this play over the next several weeks, his degree of erection started to increase noticeably and he began reporting success in terms of degrees of erection (from 0 to 90). At one point, we all had a laugh when I started a session with a typical, but in this case inappropriate, opener: "What's up this week?" He continued to report higher degrees of arousal and a sensation very much like orgasm but without ejaculation. Once again, we reviewed the idea that the point of our work was increased enjoyment and not productivity.

When he had reported substantial but not complete erection several weeks in a row (expressed as 60 to 70 degrees), we moved to the assignment of inserting his penis into her vagina without attempting intercourse. In this instance, they reported that doing so was not possible. In general, I have found that couples either can manage this easily with a moderately erect penis or cannot do it, and find the idea somewhat preposterous. Fred and his partner were in the latter category. In fact, their progress essentially plateaued at this level. They were quite happy with the improvement, and his girlfriend felt considerable relief from learning that he really was enjoying their lovemaking and pleasuring her, as well as the increase in the range of their lovemaking activity.

While we were working on this phase and realizing that progress had reached a limit, relationship issues began to surface. As is true at any age, in late life, sexual counseling is seldom only about sex. Fred began to express some concerns about the future of the relationship. His girlfriend was approaching a career change, and her husband was considering moving back into the area at about the same time. These issues prompted some very realistic concerns about whether their relationship was going to last much longer. The secrecy of their meetings was becoming more difficult to maintain. Finally, relationships tend to be dynamic and growing, and it is difficult to maintain a stable status quo, as they were attempting to do.

While these issues were aired and discussed in the couples sessions, they basically decided to continue as they were. His girlfriend was able to provide some reassurance about her intentions, but was also quite frank not only about the possibility of having to move away for career reasons but also that her estranged husband's return would reduce the frequency of their visits. Fred was able to be candid about his sense of insecurity, his jealousy about her husband's return, and a felt desire for more closeness, although he recognized the limits and felt that what they had was better than not having her in his life.

By mutual consent, the therapy ended at this point with a recognition of progress having been made, even though original goals were not achieved. Fred continued with his primary therapist. I have heard since then, via messages sent through the other therapist, that their relationship has continued at this level for several years, even though his girlfriend did move to another city a few hours' drive from Fred.

DISCUSSION

Rapport Building. Fred and I established rapport almost instantly. He was very much accustomed to therapy and had been well prepared for our visits by his principal therapist. He was a very likable man and had lived a very interesting life. My major challenge with Fred was to keep him on topic during sessions. He would at times divert the conversation onto unrelated topics. Unfortunately for me, these digressions were often extremely interesting, and it was difficult not let them go on and so waste the therapy hour.

His girlfriend was also a very intelligent and likable person with experience in counseling. She was very open about their relationship, and both of them were very open about their sexual life. In general, I have found older adults to be open and unembarrassed in discussing sexual issues. In training new therapists, it is typically the younger adult who is embarrassed, awkward, and resistant to broaching sexual issues with an older client.

Techniques in Therapy. In terms of technique as such, I have found little need to vary the basic approaches, which are used in sexual counseling with younger adults, when working with sexual dysfunction in late life. Sexual histories are, of course, longer. However, the same general problems occur in terms of performance anxiety, taking a spectator role, and so on. There is generally less need to educate people about sexuality, although there are notable exceptions. For example, one woman saw her husband's interest in fellatio with women as evidence of homosexuality. In Fred's case, the only modification was willingness to work within the context of an atypical relationship. This change points to a frequently encountered problem in working on sexuality in later life: The major problem for most older adults is the lack of suitable partners. I have interviewed at least as many older adults with sexual problems, who had no access to a regular sexual partner, as I have seen older adults in counseling specifically focused on sexuality.

Gerontological Issues. Therapists working with older adults need to be comfortable discussing sexual issues and sexual histories with the elderly. Doing so calls attention to the existence of cohort differences in sexual behavior and change in sexual behavior over time. A number of clients have commented on the increasing popularity and acceptance of oral sex as a mode of sexual expression. Older female clients have often pointed to becoming aware of their potential for orgasm during the sixties, when magazines began carrying articles on clitoral orgasm.

In terms of changes over the life span, older men tend to confirm the reports of less intense interest in sex, longer refractory periods, and a need for more stimulation to be physically aroused. Most male clients have reflected on this change as positive. Typical comments concern having more time to enjoy sex, as opposed to its "being over before you know it." Another frequent comment is that they feel relieved that sex no longer controls them, but they control their sexuality. I have also been intrigued that many men who have become physically impotent maintain active sex lives, giving pleasure to women and enjoying doing so very much.

For older women, my clients' reports suggest that the role of developmental changes seems less influential than prior experience with sex. That is, older female clients with whom I have talked seem to be divided into those who never enjoyed sex and have no interest in it and those who had pleasurable sexual experience and maintain an active interest if circumstances permit it. By far the most frequent sexual problem I have heard from older women is the lack of an acceptable partner. Older women who have a lifelong preference for a slightly older male partner, and for sex within the context of an intimate and committed marital relationship, face difficult choices between maintaining these values and life without sex.

Within marriages, the awareness of closeness to death often brings conflicts over certain sexual practices to a peak. One partner may decide that they really need to have a certain sexual experience before they die. Oral sex has been the most common issue for couples I have seen; anal intercourse and trying a specific new position for intercourse are also common. The other partner is then faced with the choice between engaging in an act that he or she may find repulsive or having his or her spouse go elsewhere. While much could be made of the symbolism or the strategic value of such "last chance" stances, they are a not uncommon source of friction in late-life marriages. If the couple's children are included in the discussion, both the alignments of children with either spouse and the children's reactions to the issue intensify the conflict and draw out long-standing family alliances and conflicts.

Relationship Issues. To my knowledge, there were no strong transferential issues evidenced in this case. My countertransferential issues surfaced in different ways twice during this relatively brief intervention. First, as has often been my experience in sexually focused counseling, I found Fred's girlfriend very attractive for three or four sessions during the therapy. Aside from some mild difficulty in concentrating on what I was saying, and a couple of interesting daydreams, there was little effect from this erotic attraction since I have enough sense and ethics to recognize and control any such impulses.

Slightly later, as the relationship issues came more to the forefront, I found myself sufficiently aligned with Fred to want to take his side and talk her into leaving her husband and making the most of the relationship with Fred. Again, I recognized the impulse for what it was and stayed focused on helping them talk about their relationship and discover what they wanted to do.

Summary. The major lesson to be learned from Fred's story is the importance of being able to talk with older adults about sex. It has been my experience that the discomfort around this topic in therapy is virtually always the younger therapist's embarrassment at talking with an older person about sexual issues. While I have had clients calmly refuse to discuss sexual issues, I have never had an older client become highly embarrassed or offended when I raised this issue.

Obviously, older adults have had more experience with their own sexuality than younger adults have. Normal change in the physiology of sexual response, and common changes in the social context for sexual behavior in later life, can produce problems; but these problems occur after decades of experience that have helped to define personal sexuality and usually bring some degree of comfortable acceptance of it. Young adults seemed convinced, contrary to all evidence and simple logic, that sex is wholly owned by the young. There is hope that Fred's story can assist in dispelling that particularly persistent myth about later life.

CHAPTER TEN

Agnes:
Living Alone With Dying

When she was first seen by our team, Agnes was in her 60s, had been widowed for more than 10 years, and was a retired buyer for a department store. Initially, she was seen by another therapist on the team for treatment of depression, which was interfering with her recovery from cancer. She had been through surgery and chemotherapy and was considered to be in remission at that time. She and her physician both felt that she was depressed and socially inactive to an extent not explainable either by the disease process or by the effects of the treatment. By working on expression of feelings, realistic expectations of treatment, and goal-setting for increased out-of-home activity and increased social activity, there was some steady improvement in her mood and her activity.

Three types of changes occurred after this initial phase of therapy. One was that the activity outside the home was often cut short because of episodes of shortness of breath and feelings of panic. Because her cancer had partly involved the respiratory system, and because of the possibility that this was a side-effect of medication, she was encouraged to discuss this with her physician, who then shared his findings with us. At this point, the conclusion was that there was no physical basis for these episodes.

Based on that conclusion, part of each therapy session revolved around teaching relaxation and structured desensitization for the sense of being short of breath. She had some difficulty with the passive relaxation, having generally preferred exercise as a method of stress reduction. Obviously, her ability to use this preferred method was curtailed by the shortness-of-breath symptom. There was modest improvement, with fewer panic episodes and a reduced intensity when they did occur; however, the shortness of breath continued, and she still avoided some activities because of this symptom.

Second, an increasing focus of therapy was her relationship with her children, especially her daughter. She felt that her daughter was not supportive enough. In fact, their relationship had generally been stormy and somewhat distant. As therapy progressed, much of her dissatisfaction with life was attributed to lack of support from her daughter, her daughter's temper, and so on. Her daughter lived in the same town and they saw each other weekly, but these visits were not satisfactory for Agnes. She was not open to family sessions with her daughter. In contrast, she had generally positive feelings about her son, who lived about 50 miles away, had her up only for visits on holidays, and rarely called her. She felt that this level of involvement was appropriate from him in that he was busy with his own family and work responsibilities, whereas her daughter was unmarried and had no children.

The third change was a recurrence of the cancer. Agnes was angry with the doctor, whom she felt had misled her and given her false hope. She felt abysmally unlucky in having a recurrence of a cancer for which recovery rates were generally high. She was depressed at this point, mainly due to the realization that surgery and chemotherapy were in her immediate future, rather than because death was near. She had had a bad experience with chemotherapy and had finished it saying "never again."

In fact, she was now quite uncertain that she wanted to go through treatment again. With support and prompting from her therapist (who in turn drew support from discussing the situation in both group and individual supervision), she had several conversations with her physician about her probable course of treatment and the likelihood of survival with and without the treatment. He was candid with her to the effect that survival was only marginally better with treatment than without. She then discussed with her therapist her feelings about surgery and chemotherapy and her ideas about quality of life versus prolonging life. After about four sessions of such discussion, she decided not to go through with the treatment.

The following week she called to cancel her appointment because she was going into the hospital for surgery. Her therapist called and visited her in the hospital to show support and caring, although Agnes was generally weak and often barely conscious. Her daughter was virtually always there and obviously quite distressed by her mother's condition. When Agnes went home, the daughter moved in with her for a while and gave her considerable personal care. As Agnes recovered, their relationship became more tense, with arguments about housekeeping and Agnes' personal care, and the daughter left after an argument. When Agnes was well enough, therapy continued with home visits and eventually moved back to the office. She had chemotherapy, but also negotiated with her physician for lower doses that left her mentally alert. These lower doses were thought to be less effective in eradicating the cancer.

About 2 months after the end of chemotherapy, Agnes was much like she had been before the recurrence. She went out as often as she could. The shortness of breath, now seen as a physical symptom, still limited her, but she could talk herself through the panic attacks and could pace herself to avoid many attacks of shortness of breath. She still focused much of her dissatisfaction with life on her daughter. She felt alone. She was angry about her second course of medical treatment and fearful that another would be needed. She remembered having decided not to pursue treatment and had not so much changed her mind as simply awakened one morning and called the doctor to schedule surgery.

The question on our minds as therapists at this point was: Did Agnes know that she would probably die within the next year or two? Should we ask her and so challenge her apparent denial? After the initial diagnosis of the recurrence of cancer, she had never again mentioned the probable limiting of her life to a period ranging from several months to a couple of years. After some discussion with the entire outreach team, it was decided to at least raise the question and give her the opportunity to talk about and prepare for her death. It was felt that her relationship with her daughter in particular represented a large piece of unfinished business and that she should have the chance to decide what she wanted to do about not only that but also the rest of her life.

When the question was broached, it appeared that she was aware of the likely limit on her life. She had felt that the therapist would be as uncomfortable discussing this issue as she felt her daughter was. She agreed that the situation with her daughter was a major problem for her, but also felt that it was unresolvable. She continued to assert that her daughter would never come in for therapy and would not change even if she did. Her therapist challenged her perceptions of her daughter's uncaring stance by reminding her of her daughter's support during the illness, but Agnes dismissed that. We became convinced that there was some long-standing issue between them, and also that we would likely never discover what it was.

At this time, the individual therapy appeared to become stuck, and Agnes was referred to a therapy group that I was starting. Agnes was a quiet group member, supportive of the others and only occasionally talking about herself. She would sometimes smile quietly to herself as one of the others would talk at length about physical symptoms that resulted in anxiety but were neither disabling nor life-threatening. Asked by a third member to comment on her feelings about listening to these complaints, she quite diplomatically acknowledged that everyone is most concerned about their own pain, and that nearing death had given her a different perspective, so that her arthritis pains were now almost a welcome reminder that she was still alive. The group was supportive and listened when she did talk about preparing for death, bringing up examples of loved ones who had died and what they had done and said about approaching death.

Another group member's story about a dysfunctional daughter prompted Agnes to discuss her own daughter's struggles with drugs (she was now drug free) and with mental disorder. Her daughter had been hospitalized a few times as a young woman and now led a fairly normal life on medication. Agnes felt disappointed and guilty about her daughter's life and was resentful that her daughter's inability to tolerate stress meant that she was less available to Agnes. Other group members responded with accounts of their own families, which made it clear that Agnes was not alone and, in fact, had more support and contact with her children than most other group members. Drawing on their own experience, a couple of members pointed out that Agnes's disappointment in her daughter could be a major part of the strain between them. If this was understood, it had no obvious impact over time.

In a spontaneous effort to get her life in order and prepare for death, Agnes made plans to go back to New York City and visit her siblings and her mother, who had recently been placed in a nursing home there. For whatever reason, it came as a surprise to us that she had relatives in the East and that her brothers and her mother were living. She had only talked about her life in California, which spanned several decades.

Before the trip she reminisced about growing up in New York and about places she wanted to see again. She expressed considerable concern about her mother's condition and her brother's decision to place their mother in a nursing home. As near as she knew, her mother had a multi-infarct dementia, which had worsened over time. After the trip, she reported good childhood memories and recollections of places she had not seen in years. She had accepted her mother's placement since she was nearly nonverbal and barely seemed to recognize Agnes.

Agnes had been fearful that her mother would die before she had a chance to visit again and felt finished with that. She also discussed her relationship with her mother, which had been stormy, and that she had always felt her mother disapproved of her. She had moved to California in part to put distance between them. The parallels to her relationship with her own daughter were acknowledged, but seemed to increase her sense of the inevitability of the problem. In fact, the group tended to reinforce this feeling with their nearly unanimous experience of feeling closer to their sons, of whom they expected little, and being disappointed in and somewhat alienated from rebellious daughters.

This trip and her sense of completion with her mother and brothers seemed to achieve a sense of acceptance of dying for Agnes. She continued to come to group and work on control of her panic episodes (currently redefined yet again as psychogenic, rather than biomedical in origin) and on being clear in her requests of her daughter and realistic in her expectations of that relationship.

I left that group while she was continuing to work on these day-to-day issues.

DISCUSSION

Rapport Building. Agnes accepted me readily enough as a therapist, and our relationship remained professional and role-determined throughout the time we worked together. She is representative of the many older clients I have seen for shorter periods of time, in that our relationship was relatively easy in its beginning and never became especially deep or complex.

Techniques in Therapy. Agnes received considerable training in relaxation and in the use of cognitive strategies to control her anxiety. This approach is generally helpful with people who are short of breath and anxious about it, since the anxiety tends to exacerbate the shortness of breath. For people who are able to use relaxation, the technique tends to disrupt the upward spiral of breathing problems causing anxiety, which causes more trouble breathing, and so on. The use of relaxation tends to be helpful whether the problem is physical or psychological in origin. Emphasizing this fact avoids becoming entangled in debates about whether the problem is psychological in the sense of being less real or "all in my head," which is a common form of resistance. Also, as was true in Agnes's case, it is often unclear how much of the problem is determined by physical or psychological causes.

Much of the work with Agnes focused on encouraging her to explore her feelings and talk about her life in preparation for dying. This type of therapy is often quite simple from the standpoint of technique because it mainly involves skillful and sustained listening (Kübler-Ross, 1969; Rando, 1984). At the same time, it appears to be very difficult work because very few people seem to be able or willing to sit and listen. Often a focus on "unfinished business" will emerge, and so, as with Agnes, use of family systems perspectives and other therapeutic approaches may emerge as important. In her case, much of this work was accomplished by a trip to New York, which was perhaps occasioned by therapy but certainly was not planned in therapy.

Gerontological Issues. Agnes introduces several phenomena that are fairly common aspects of working with older adults. The concern that perhaps she did not know that her condition was immediately terminal, or that perhaps denial was the best coping strategy for her, is rather typical of discussions about introducing the topic of preparation for dying into therapy. Also typical is the outcome: Agnes was quite aware of the nearness of death and much more comfortable discussing it than her therapists were. In fact, she had been protecting us, both accurately perceiving our discomfort and also incorrectly assuming that we would be as uncomfortable with the topic as her daughter was.

It is also worthy of note that her response to discussing whether to continue treatment is also common, though certainly not universal. She explored the options with her therapist, reached the decision that she did not want to continue the cancer treatment while she was in therapy, and then went home and changed her mind. I have so often seen people go through this process of making careful decisions and then changing their minds, frequently more than once, that I am somewhat suspicious of reports of decision making about continuing or discontinuing life that do not evidence some ambivalence.

People, including therapists and family members, can have strongly held convictions about the decision and can have an even stronger need for the decision process to be concluded and stay concluded. I suspect that some individuals wrestling with this issue are overtly or covertly influenced, by those with whom they talk, to decide a certain way or to stick to a decision once it is made. It would seem that the decision to die, or to increase or decrease one's risk of death and the quality of one's remaining life, is such a uniquely personal and important decision that it needs to be made without influence from those around us.

The ambiguity about whether Agnes's breathing problems were physical or psychological is rather typical of work with psychosomatic symptoms in later life. The determination is often difficult to impossible to make, and it is not uncommon that the physician or physicians involved will change their minds over the course of time. The therapist needs to be able to tolerate this ambiguity and also to formulate interventions that are likely to help in either case or at least will not interfere with medical treatment, should it turn out that the problem is physiological after all. These are not inconsequential guidelines: Many psychotherapists and other psychosocial workers are sufficiently negative about medical practice that they convey to the client that medicines are not necessary, that further diagnosis would be inappropriate, and so on.

Another aspect of Agnes's therapy that is frequent in work with the elderly is the emergence of new family members after several months in therapy. Whether this is due to the tendency of younger professionals to assume that the elderly are isolated and alone in the world, or whether clients often conceal or neglect to mention the existence of some family members for emotionally motivated reasons, is unclear to me. In Agnes's case, it would seem she had neglected to mention the New York relatives because of her emotional distance from them and because of her ambivalence about seeing her mother again with the fear that she would die before she had the opportunity to do so.

Relationship Issues. Agnes's relationship to me seemed relatively uncomplicated by relationship distortions. As I write this, I find myself wondering if some of the distance that I discussed in regard to rapport was not due to my protecting myself from the experience of getting close to yet another client who would die soon. While I have generally been able to be quite open with dying clients, I do have the perception that it was difficult to maintain this openness over time. The time in my life when I saw Agnes was especially trying for me, and I may very well have been holding back to some extent for self-protection. To be fair, Agnes was also fairly emotionally distanced from her own family members, and so I may simply be experiencing the remoteness that she maintained with everyone.

Summary. As was true for the previous case discussion about sexuality in late life, perhaps the major therapeutic issue in working with older adults who are dying is being able to ask them about their feelings about death and to listen to what they say. There is no other therapeutic work that is easier conceptually and technically. Much of the time one is engaged in active listening and in keeping one's mouth shut while watching another human being struggle with the types of questions and feelings that baffle and frighten all of us.

Especially as I have become involved in training new therapists, it has become more obvious to me over the years that this simple work is extraordinarily difficult for most people. Knowing the right things to do is not readily translated into action. Driven by anxiety about dying, most of us will avoid the topic, avoid the probing for feelings, and say the wrong things or simply say too much (cf. Lehman, Ellard, & Wortman, 1986; Peters-Golden, 1982).

Oddly, little training is provided on this most difficult topic in psychotherapy, and even less is of the experiential sort that will help the therapist identify and work through personal blind spots regarding death and dying issues. Much more consideration should be given to providing support for therapists and other professional helpers who regularly face death and dying in their work. Frequent confrontation with death may well be a factor in burn-out in working with the elderly in all settings.

CHAPTER ELEVEN

Jerry and Bea:
Preparation for Dying, a Marital Case

Our first contact with Jerry and Bea was Bea's call requesting therapy for her husband, whom she saw as depressed and not handling retirement and aging at all well. Even on the telephone, it seemed clear that Bea herself was in considerable distress, with anxiety and hostility apparent. She was quite definite that Jerry was the person with the problem, although she was equally clear that he would not see it that way.

In the initial interview, Jerry was quiet, reserved, and unemotional, while Bea was highly verbal and intense. Jerry was clearly there at her insistence, but was willing to try therapy. They were both in their early 60s. Jerry had been retired for 3 years and had become active in a local volunteer organization and, through that group, in local politics. He had been an engineer in a large defense contractor company. Bea had worked in clerical and bookkeeping positions and had volunteered for years in counseling-related projects. She had taken community college level classes in psychology and counseling and clearly felt as competent as the two therapists working with herself and her husband. They had moved from a suburban Los Angeles County neighborhood into a Ventura County senior citizen mobile home park, whose residents had an average age in the 80s.

Presenting problems basically centered on activities and communication. Jerry was seen as overinvolved in his separate activities and not sufficiently available for household chores and joint couples activities. He was seen (by Bea) as not supportive enough of her, incommunicative, and having trouble adjusting to retirement. He presented himself as feeling fine except for having too many arguments at home. We concluded this initial assessment by urging that they both become clients and recommending that we see them separately, with regular conjoint sessions involving both therapists and the couple.

We proceeded on this basis for a few weeks. Separately, Bea was more overtly angry, both about Jerry and at the therapist, a young male social worker, whom she frequently criticized and second-guessed. Jerry was somewhat more open about himself and more open about the importance of their arguments in his life, although he remained skeptical about the likelihood that therapy would help. Exploring this skepticism, which was at first presented as part of his general worldview as an older man and an engineer, revealed that they had previously had therapy.

About 10 years earlier, Bea had become involved in a project to help youth at risk of becoming juvenile offenders. She received training in counseling and became very attached to the professor who ran the project. Jerry was uncertain if the involvement was romantic, but the intensity was similar. She entered individual therapy and decided that she and Jerry needed to separate. Their children had left home, and she felt they needed to reevaluate the relationship. He moved into an apartment and fairly quickly found a girlfriend. When the girlfriend was ready to move in with him, Bea decided it was time for reconciliation.

They began living together again and started seeing Bea's therapist (also a middle-aged woman) as a couple. Jerry felt that the two of them had tended to "gang up" on him and he had responded by being stubborn and quiet in the sessions. He felt the therapy had done no good. He was also unable to say why he and Bea had stayed together in an unchanged relationship.

At about this point, they arrived for a conjoint session, with Bea looking extremely fatigued and ill. Questioning revealed that she was "back on chemotherapy" and was having considerable problems with nausea. This was our first hint that Bea was having any problem with cancer. In this session, it came out that she had had a successful mastectomy at about the time they reunited from the separation described above. She had been in remission for several years, but a recurrence, which had metastasized by the time of diagnosis, had recently been discovered. She was on chemotherapy, with considerable side-effects and a very uncertain prognosis.

Being astute clinicians, we suggested that perhaps her illness was having some impact on each of them and on their relationship. We also expressed surprise and concern that they had not even mentioned the illness before now. Bea felt that her years in support groups for women with mastectomy and her experience as a hospice volunteer counselor had prepared her for this situation and that she was handling it fine. Jerry professed to see no connection between her illness and any problems they had.

However, starting with the next visit, the focus shifted to her illness. She felt angry that her nearly textbook recovery from breast cancer had shifted to undetected recurrence and metastasis with a very uncertain prognosis. She felt that Jerry and her children were insufficiently supportive and that his outside activities were a distraction from her illness. He expressed concern about her illness, fear of losing her, and frustration with her frequent noncompliance with treatment and her continued involvement in community groups and college classes. It developed at this point that she, too, was very involved and often pushed herself to continue in activities when obviously overtired or nauseated. He reported that she often came home and went to bed for several hours.

In both individual and conjoint sessions, the therapeutic work took on the dual focus of acknowledging and communicating feelings about the progression of the illness and the possibility of Bea's death on one hand, and behavioral change focused on increasing time together and decreasing destructive arguments on the other. Bea was able to express her frustration with physicians, the treatment, and Jerry quite easily. She was also disappointed in the lack of response from her children, especially from a son who was a minister. It was unclear whether the children had been plainly told of her condition, and attempts to arrange sessions with the children when they came to visit were always blocked. She also frequently criticized us for the way we responded to her.

A critical turning point for her was a session in which we all discussed the pros and cons of chemotherapy for her. She eventually concluded that she would refuse future rounds of chemotherapy since there was no clear indication of progress in treating the cancer and the chemotherapy clearly made her fatigued and nauseous. The session concluded with a clear sense of accomplishment and closure around a very difficult issue. When she returned the following week, she was back on chemotherapy and feeling modestly hopeful about the likelihood of successful treatment.

Jerry was gradually able to express his sense of helplessness in the face of the illness and his sadness about the possibility of losing Bea. He teared up at times but never cried. He was also very concerned about her high level of activity and consequent exhaustion, as well as the arguments that frequently accompanied her fatigue. In conjoint sessions, by active intervention including editing, dictating whose turn it was to speak, and prompting each to discuss areas that had been agreed upon in individual sessions, we were able to increase communication of feelings.

By negotiation and behavioral prescription, they were able to slightly decrease time in individual activities. Jerry became more involved in housework. He never seemed to feel okay about this, even when it was clear that she was increasingly unable to do more difficult chores. She was constantly critical of his efforts in this direction. There was a modest impact on arguments. They were able to recognize, and at times avoid, situations that often led to arguments. They were not able to see what each contributed to arguments or to conceptualize the arguments as "scripts" or "games." Each remained very involved in who was right and who was wrong in every argument. Since there was very little progress in behavior change, my cotherapist encouraged them to see the arguments as one of their mutually shared activities.

A review of the history of their relationship gave both of them a clearer perspective on why they were together. Bea's father had left her at an early age, and then her mother died when Bea was in her teens. While in high school she lived with an aunt's family who provided for her, but did not provide a sense of being wanted. She was out and working on her own immediately after graduation from high school, and met Jerry through his cousin who was dating a friend of hers. They dated a few weeks and married. He was seen by her then as much more mature and settled. He had a steady job and his unemotional demeanor suggested stability and security at that time.

Jerry saw himself as being from a very average background with a happy childhood. He had been shy throughout school and college and had seldom dated. Bea was the most attractive girl he had met, and he had seen her as vivacious and exciting. This brief review not only served as a reminder of the historical basis of their relationship but also could be used to show the positive side of traits and themes that had later become irritating.

Therapy ended not by mutual agreement, but by a series of missed appointments and Bea and Jerry's gradual withdrawal. The attempts to change their activities were sometimes seen as successful, but often led to resentment of things given up and charges and countercharges of noncompliance with agreements. Bea almost never admitted to perceiving changes in Jerry and remained overtly critical of our efforts to help them.

Several months later another staff member at the clinic spoke on our services to the local hospice organization. She returned to report that Bea had been there (as a volunteer counselor) and had taken the floor after the presentation to give an extensive commentary on how wonderful our services were and how much help we had been to her personally in coping with her illness. We were astonished at this report.

A few months after that we read Bea's obituary in the local paper.

DISCUSSION

Rapport Building. Bea and Jerry are an example of working with clients with whom one never does establish rapport. It is quite questionable whether we ever established a clear sense of working together in the therapy. Jerry was always somewhat reserved and questioning the value of being there; Bea was challenging us at every turn. In fact, until we heard of her later public endorsement of us, we had assumed that she considered the therapy to have failed her.

We (the two therapists) had numerous talks during the therapy about this apparent lack of basic rapport. In general, we were constantly trying to decide whether to continue the therapy or tell them that we simply were not getting anywhere. We continued because they kept coming in and kept working with us, even though the work was clearly difficult and even though they verbally simultaneously expressed considerable doubt and lack of commitment.

Jerry's ambivalence was clearly a combination of his background in a more concrete, problem-solving occupation, where results could be seen, and seen quickly, along with his previous highly negative experiences with therapy as a competitor that was taking his wife away from him. Bea's ambivalence was the combination of conflict between her emerging identity with a mid-life career in counseling and being in therapy with younger and more fully trained men, along with a basic struggle over whether she would confront her problems. Although the more obviously emotionally distressed and the one with terminal illness, Bea called originally to get help for Jerry and continued to displace her distress onto him. She also denied her illness so completely that it came up in therapy only when the effects of the chemotherapy made it unavoidable as a topic. We decided that to insist on a clear verbal commitment, and a clear feeling on our part that we had rapport, would be equivalent to denying therapy to this needy couple.

Although Bea and Jerry are an extreme example, there is a general phenomenon in therapy with older adults that this example illustrates. In general, it seems to me that in working with older adults, one has to rely more on their behavioral compliance with therapy than on what is said about the therapeutic endeavor as an indicator of commitment to therapy. Older adults often approach therapy with a more experimental and more judgmental attitude, as compared to younger adults, who may be more ready to believe that therapy will solve their problems and more willing to become dependent on the therapist.

If one is accustomed to, or needs, a fair amount of verbal approval from clients and a sense that clients are committed in the sense of being dependent, working with older adults may provide less of this than does work with younger adults. Based on clinical experience, this difference may influence the therapist's sense of comfort or confidence, but does not seem to dramatically affect the outcome of the therapeutic work: I've felt quite connected to clients who changed very little, and have had little sense of rapport with clients who changed greatly.

Techniques in Therapy. The primary focus of technique in working with Bea and Jerry was a communication skills enhancement (cf. Gottman et al., 1976). They were clearly not communicating well and just as clearly not compromising on issues where they were in disagreement. Although Bea was more verbal and had enough training to frame her speech in psychotherapy talk, she was not talking about what really mattered to her any more than Jerry was. While she talked a lot, she mainly talked about his problems and talked in fairly abstract psychological terminology. She was not talking about what it felt like to face death, what she wanted from him, what her fears were, and so on. He, on the other hand, simply quit talking altogether when things got uncomfortable. They were able, over a period of a few months, to change much of this pattern. First, each of them put feelings into words and clear requests in the individual meetings. The next steps were to practice these changes with one another in conjoint meetings and, finally, with one another at home.

There was also need for negotiation of compromises. Both wanted more time together, but each was involved in numerous outside activities. This actually came to light as Jerry cut back on his commitments to spend more time at home, only to discover that Bea was not there because of her commitments. At that point, Bea had to decide to cut back on some of her classes and social commitments if she really wanted more time with her husband.

The review of the history of their relationship was also helpful in gaining perspective on current difficulties. Remembering why they got together, and seeing the similarities between what had attracted them in the beginning and the polarities that were now irritating, provided a healthy sense of perspective of "the cup is half full" variety.

The key, and most difficult, topic for communication was the fact of her approaching death. It was on both their minds, but there had been no communication at all about it. It had become a family secret and a major block in their communication. This type of block in talking about dying is not at all unusual but is still destructive of relationships, even though often maintained for good reasons. In working with a self-help group for cancer patients several years ago, we found it necessary to separate the patients and the spouses into different rooms, and talk separately, before talking together could become a possibility (Wollert, Knight, & Levy, 1980).

Similarly with Bea and Jerry, we discussed it with each of them separately and then had both of them discuss it together. They were both genuinely surprised that the other had thought so much about it and that each had real concerns about the effect of the situation on the other. That is, he was quite worried about her dying, how much she would suffer, and how much she was pushing herself to maintain a high level of activity, which frequently left her exhausted and depressed. She was worried about his ability to handle the emotional impact of losing her and also about his ability to take care of himself after she was gone (cooking, cleaning, and so on). Both were quite touched by the mutual concern. The sharing led to some change in the way they were living day-to-day, primarily in increasing their motivation to spend time together.

Gerontological Issues. Bea and Jerry are prime examples of a couple in denial about the approach of death. Perhaps our greatest contribution to their relationship was getting them to talk to one another about their feelings about Bea's dying. This goal was primarily ours, rather than theirs, in its initiation. That is, we were quite active in encouraging them to talk about her dying in individual sessions and in setting it as a goal for the couple's sessions. We had no agenda for what needed to be said, but it was clearly our agenda that they needed to say something to one another before she died.

This stance comes from a concern with preparation for dying that is a key issue in learning about later life, and also from work with many widows and widowers who feel incomplete for exactly this reason: Nothing was said or settled before the death. Death is an ultimate reality and of ultimate importance in life and is perhaps the only event in relationships that cannot be undone or redone. Conversations with a dying person that are put off too long simply never happen. For these reasons, counseling with dying individuals and their families is one of the few times when it becomes permissible to give direct advice about the importance of talking about it and saying things you have always wanted to say.

We have found often, however, that therapists unacquainted with preparation for dying work can miss the issue entirely. Bea and Jerry illustrate how this might happen: They were in significant denial and never really volunteered information about her cancer. The conversation that led to their revealing it was started by the therapist, who commented on how weak and ill Bea looked, pressed for reasons, and then concluded that this was a topic that needed pursuing. Even when death and dying issues arise, some therapists feel comfortable accepting the clients' assurance that this is not really a problem, or may even rationalize that denial is the best and most appropriate defense in such circumstances.

Having said that, one can also note that there is a danger in having many, if any, convictions about what decisions need to be made or what needs to be talked about. The whole topic of decision making about death, right to die, right to refuse treatment, and so on is a highly charged and value-laden topic. Most people tend to have strong ideas and feelings on this issue, and it becomes exactly the kind of topic where the therapist's (or other helper's) values and feelings may influence the outcome of the client's decision making. At the same time and for the same reasons, it is exactly the kind of topic on which therapist and client may disagree and for which the client's values need to take priority. To the fullest extent possible, the therapist needs to restrict herself or himself to the task of facilitating the process of the decision making, without influencing the content of that decision. While we each tend to have opinions that we are clear about for ourselves, we need only contemplate what it would mean to unduly influence someone else's decision and be wrong to understand why it is important to maintain a standard of working only with the process.

Experience with such counseling has reinforced this position for me in two ways. First, I have seen people content with both kinds of decisions and I have also seen people unhappy with both kinds of decisions. Experience has taught me that I have no idea what will work for someone else. Second, as illustrated by Agnes in the preceding example and by Bea in this one, people quite frequently change their minds. The decision is so complex, and the implications so far-reaching, that many people have to decide one way for a while, and live with that for a few days, to realize that they really want to make the other decision. Obviously, enthusiastic endorsement of a given decision by others may make it difficult for a person to change his or her mind again.

The decision is perhaps roughly comparable to the complexity of deciding whether to stay in a distressed marriage: The decision to seek a divorce may be the first step toward divorce or may be a step toward reevaluating the marriage; thinking about leaving may remind the client about what is good about the marriage. Friends or a therapist, who, for their own reasons, would like to see the client get divorced may make changing one's mind more difficult. Similarly, deciding not to seek treatment and dying a natural death can, for some, be a first step toward making a decision to hold on to life.

In summary, deciding whether to continue active treatment, which has serious side effects that dramatically reduce the quality of one's life for the short period left, is clearly a highly individualized decision that ought to be made free of outside influence. Our clinical observation is that this decision-making process is complex and fragile in the sense that decisions are often made and later reversed. In general, everyone with whom the dying person interacts will have strong convictions and feelings on the matter. Many professional helpers will also be employed by an agency or institution that has a policy on the decision to die (e.g., hospitals may require active participation in treatment if one remains in hospital; hospice services may require a consistent decision to die naturally). The principle, that one should facilitate the process of making the decision without influencing the actual decision, will be profoundly more difficult to practice than to state.

Relationship Issues. Perhaps the essential aspect of Bea and Jerry's relationship to us was their general disposition toward us as therapists. Bea had the conflict of comparing herself as a counselor to us and needing to see herself as better. She also compared us, as the younger, unavailable males, with the middle-aged professor, who had introduced her to counseling and for whom she clearly had romantic feelings as well as high regard as a counselor and mentor. Combined with her ambivalence about confronting the central issues in her life, these comparisons blocked the development of a normally positive relationship with us as therapists.

Jerry was caught up in comparison with a past negative experience, in which he perceived therapists as ganging up on him. He also tended to see therapy as women's work. This view was part of the worldview associated with his stereotypically masculine work role and was part of his life experience. Therapy had been something that Bea did and something she got him involved with—and with a woman therapist. Not inclined to be emotionally expressive or very communicative to begin with, he was not encouraged by these past experiences to see therapy as a positive force in his life.

From our side, we were confronted with two clients who kept coming in and working, but were somewhat difficult to work with and clearly did not like us or respect us very much. It was difficult not to get engaged in Bea's challenges to our method or styles, as opposed to staying focused on her use of these challenges to avoid doing therapeutic work. The discovery that she was dying and avoiding talking about it made her a more sympathetic person for us. It was much more difficult to accept the resistance without knowing what was being suppressed.

As we became more sympathetic to her and learned more about her life, the fact of her approaching death became sadder. She clearly had rarely been close to anyone in her life and had tended to push people away. While she improved her relationship with Jerry, they were still not very close and she had, in our view, significant unfinished business with her children. She clearly had very little time to work on such issues, and also very little inclination to do so, even as she felt the loneliness of approaching death with relatively little support from family and friends.

We have very little indication as to what happened after she left therapy. Clearly she coped in part by getting involved in hospice as a helper rather than as a client, a stance that would be consistent with her struggles with us. We were left with the sense of incompletion that often comes with clients who drift away from therapy and with the knowledge that she would die in the near future with many issues unresolved. There is considerable sadness in that kind of ending with a client.

Summary. The work with Bea and Jerry helps to illustrate the indirect way in which death and dying issues may arise in psychotherapy. Their presenting complaint was about marital interaction, and even in discussing their communication problems, there was tacit agreement between the two of them not to discuss Bea's approaching death. The work with them was a blend of couple's communication skills enhancement and preparation for dying counseling. In effect, we had to improve their ability to communicate so that they could talk about her dying.

The ending of their therapy also illustrates vividly the higher stakes that one often confronts in working with older adults. In other situations where I have been less than successful with a client, there is the hope that they will either try again with someone else or in some other way find a solution to the problem that they are struggling with. With Bea it was quite clear that there was no future that allowed for alternate solutions. While I do not feel responsible for her refusal to use therapy, there is an absolute finality in her refusal that is not present with other clients who terminate.

CHAPTER TWELVE

Nora:
Physical Symptoms as Substitutes for Emotion

Nora was in her early 60s, married, and overweight. Retired from clerical work in various schools, she had recently moved to California from New York City. She made an appointment and came in to announce that she had some problems from stress that had been made worse by her move and wanted some help and wanted it fast. She also bargained for a reduced rate of pay, based on having separate finances from her husband, but wanted me to know immediately that her marriage was not part of the problem.

When asked to describe the problem, she related that she had been told several years before that she suffered from a lot of stress. She had seen a couple of therapists very briefly (fewer than six sessions) and "gotten some advice," and had taken classes and weekend workshops on stress, assertiveness, and so on at community colleges. She still experienced her stress in physical terms and treated the more psychological explanations she had been given as "what these people told me about it." Her descriptions of the original incidents in New York sounded like panic attacks; the first occurred when she had to be anesthetized for a hysterectomy. Others related to emergency room visits for what she had thought were heart problems, but for which no physical findings emerged.

Her current stressors were fairly clear cut. She had been retired for more than a year, and her husband had taken a job in California so they could move a few years prior to his retirement. It was unclear at this point whether the decision to move was mutual, but it was quite clear that she was ambivalent about the move now that it was completed. She had two daughters, both living in the East. She was now worried about seeing them less and not being as involved with the grandchildren. She and her husband had been socially active as well as active in a Conservative Temple in New York. She was rapidly getting involved in activities through senior centers and community groups, but missed the quality of the friendships she had back East. Her husband seemed less inclined to socialize in California. The local Jewish community was Reform and "much less religious" than she was used to.

Although Nora was bright, assertive, and verbally facile, there were two types of questions that left her baffled and nearly speechless: "How do you feel about this?" and "What do you want to do?" Her reactions were phrased in terms of trouble sleeping, overeating, and "feeling stressed," which meant either muscle tension, fatigue, and upset stomach or else feeling overwhelmed by all the activities she had committed herself to.

In response to her question, "What can you do for me and how fast can you do it?" I described a plan of identifying stressors, learning to recognize her feelings more clearly, and learning to reduce distress in her life. I also told her that I was unsure how long it would take, but I was certain it would be more than the four or five visits she had allotted to other therapists. She responded by stating that she didn't have the time or the money for years of therapy. I replied that I didn't think it would take years, but more like 6 months to 2 years. Our payment structure made the number of sessions within a year irrelevant. I urged her to think about whether she really wanted therapy and to commit to at least 6 months if she did. I argued that after 6 months there would likely be noticeable improvement, if there was going to be any, and that the work of therapy would be clear to her at that time.

Her response to this was a kind of unhappy but intrigued respect. She clearly wanted a quick fix, but understood what I said and respected my description of what I thought was needed versus what she was asking for. She would allude back to our initial discussion several times in the future, with the comment that no one else had told her this in the beginning.

Our next session focused on devising strategies to control her stress. She refused progressive relaxation on the grounds that previous attempts had made her extremely uncomfortable. This seemed to be consistent with her panic attack during the early part of anesthesia. We then worked on defining what the major stressors in her life were. She described trouble sleeping, living in cramped temporary quarters, being overcommitted to activities, and problems finding a good doctor. There was a plan to get into better living quarters, which, like all such plans, was taking longer than expected. Her problems with her current physician sounded well within the range of "getting acquainted issues"; however, she had already changed doctors once in her 3 months in the community.

In short, we decided to focus on her sleeping difficulties and her tendency to overcommit to activities. We got a consent to get her medical records and to talk with her physician. His assessment was that her anxiety and her sleeping problems were emotional and not related to either her physical problems or any medication she was taking.

Over the next several months, we explored each of the issues in every session. Her overcommitment was a regular topic. We would go through problem-solving strategies and discuss each activity in terms of what she gave to it and what was either stressful or rewarding about each involvement. On several occasions, she would decide to eliminate specific activities that were stressful. This reduction in demands would reduce her stress level for a while, but she would then volunteer for more activity. Two patterns emerged during this time. First, the activities she defined as stressful usually included some element of conflict or competition with people she found distasteful. Second, during times of lessened social commitments outside the home, she would begin to share stressful interactions with family: her husband, her daughters, and a sister who lived nearby. It began to seem obvious that her activities helped her to escape from thinking about family issues.

Her sleeping problems were also a common theme during these early months. After she had kept a diary for some time, it became clear that her frequent awakening was motivated in large part by fear of heart problems. She would awaken in the night very concerned with chest pains, racing heart, and so on. She would get up, calm herself down, have a midnight snack, and write or think by herself for an hour or so, and return to sleep. She also had a regular pattern of taking naps in the afternoon. Using behavioral prescriptions to try to change these patterns (eliminating snacks and naps) improved her sleeping slightly, but mostly clarified how much she enjoyed this time to herself at night and how important her afternoon naps were to her.

Her concern over the physical sensations in her chest (and the medical assurance that there was no objective medical evidence of heart disease) led me to suspect that there was some emotional equivalent that she could acknowledge only in physical terms. We used Gendlin's (1978) focusing technique to have her identify feelings and visual images associated with the physical sensations that she interpreted as heart trouble. During focusing, the feelings were localized more in her throat than in her chest.

Since she was unable to name an emotion for the sensation at all, I threw out various alternatives. Sadness and anxiety were rejected; however, the suggestion that perhaps it was related to holding back on words she couldn't say struck a chord with her. She was very uncomfortable with the suggestion that these might be angry or even "irritated" words.

At this point, we had reached the end of our initial "trial period." Throughout this time, Nora had occasionally expressed impatience with the slowness of therapy, and I gave her the feedback that things were moving about as fast as they ever do. I also had reminded her of our agreement to see what 6 months could do. At this time we stopped and reviewed progress to date. She had, in fact, experienced some reduction in average level of distress, although she was still quite pressured and stressed. She had gained some increased awareness of her ability to control stress (i.e., she now knew that she could get out of activities), but saw from experience that she tended to increase the external stress on her own.

My point of view was that we had mainly redefined her problems: From her original sense of having several unconnected problems due to external stress, it now appeared to me that there was evidence of avoiding confrontation in her group activities, using group activities to avoid family-based issues, and perhaps a more general avoidance of anger that was worsening her perceived health and interfering with sleep. It was my thought that either she could stop where she was or we could agree to work longer on these more abstract problems.

After two or three sessions discussing what to expect if we continued further, she agreed to pursue these more abstract issues for another year. In many ways, this was the moment at which she really became engaged in the therapeutic process. She became more self-disclosing and much less teasing-questioning about the nature of therapy.

Almost immediately she told me that one reason she was reluctant to acknowledge feelings was that she had a sister who was schizophrenic and had spent her life in psychiatric hospitals and residential care homes. There was also a brother who was considered alcoholic and "unlucky in life" and had been in and out of psychiatric hospitals before dying at an early age. Both had been characterized as "emotional and sensitive" in a family that valued common sense and rationality.

Rather early in life, Nora had absorbed the implicit idea that emotionality led to craziness and, in fact, was still worried about the possibility of becoming schizophrenic. Some explanation of thought disorder, the rate of heritability in schizophrenia, the usual timing of first onsets, and questioning about her own experience of hallucinations (none) reassured her on this point.

Considerable discussion of her relationship with a surviving sister revealed years of conflict that continued into the present. During every visit, they would disagree about something and get into a heated argument about who was right and who was wrong. For example, her sister criticized her relationship with her husband, whom the sister saw as ignorant and dominating.

These disagreements were easy to start since the sisters were nearly polar opposites and always had been. Nora was more conventional, family-oriented, and religious; her sister was bohemian, single, and agnostic. In an early, symbolic incident, Nora related that after an argument in their teens, her sister had cut up her report cards and she had cut up her sister's underwear: "We each went after what was important to the other." After reviewing the history of the relationship, Nora decided to cease trying to turn their relationship into an ideal sisterly love.

Numerous incidents involved her relationship with her daughters. She felt rejected by them, even though she was the one who moved. In fact, Nora had planned and argued for the move even as the daughter who had children was urging her to move to their neighborhood. She felt the daughters should visit more often, even though it was clear that work commitments, and the fact that she and her husband lived in a small mobile home, would make visiting very difficult. Telephone interactions tended to leave Nora feeling insufficiently cared for.

We used role plays and Nora's detailed reporting of such conversations to get a better sense of how she related to her daughters. My emphasis was to explore and expand her ability to take the perspective of her daughters in their interactions. It became clear that she found anything they said inadequate to solve her problems and tended to cut them off when they tried to discuss their own troubles. In fact, at least since their teen years, it appeared that she had sought nurturance from them rather than offering it to them. This feedback was offered to her in the context of her own lifelong search for more caring and attention than was available in a large family in the early Depression years.

Her daughters had also encouraged her to be more assertive with her husband. Since all roads seemed to lead back to him, we began to discuss her relationship with her husband. She was reluctant to discuss her marriage with me, expressing the fear that therapeutic reevaluation of their marriage would lead to divorce. Her dating experience was limited to chaperoned USO dances during World War II, while she was living in a cloistered YWCA that allowed no male visitors. In spite of this protection, she had felt sexually threatened by any male attention. Her husband courted her patiently and without threatening her. A virgin when they married, she had enjoyed sex moderately until her 50s, when they discovered female orgasm by reading magazine articles describing sex research and the sexual revolution.

She described her husband as dominating, even though the history of their relationship suggested that he adapted to her increased assertiveness and her pursuit of a college education, and that most major decisions were mutual. He could be very verbally critical and loudly angry when upset. He also sometimes came home from work and cooked dinner.

Although it seemed that couples' sessions would be beneficial, she reported that he would never consider the idea and that she would not dare ask him. Some specific problems (getting some repairs around the house done) seemed to be resolved easily by her assertive requests. Her fears reduced to more manageable proportions by exploring the reality of them: Would she divorce him under any circumstances? Could she really imagine herself as a promiscuous divorcée? The concept from Kelly's personal construct theory (1955), that fear of extreme change to the polar opposite of a construct dimension inhibits more limited change, was also useful with Nora: In her case, fear of divorce kept her from making smaller scale changes in their relationship and from thinking through what postretirement marriage with her husband was going to be like.

While exploring these issues, her descriptions of interactions at her social activities continued to provide data for the concept that her symptoms were substitutes for irritation/frustration. When she was attacked or her ideas were questioned, she would become bored, sleepy, or ill and need to leave early or withdraw into another room. On one occasion, when a motion she made was challenged by another committee member, she fell asleep at the table. Her husband awakened her and took her home, expressing considerable embarrassment.

Over these months, her physical symptoms and sense of stress lessened and were replaced by anxiety and more directly experienced irritation with others. In common with other older women clients, she never endorsed the idea that she became *angry*, only *irritated*. She settled down to a relationship with one physician and to a set of social commitments that she stayed with for months at a time. She joined a discussion group that I led at a senior center, and we would debrief some of her interactions there. These sessions mainly gave her an appreciation of how she looked strong in group interactions while feeling very vulnerable.

Not long after this, a combination of change in departmental policy and in her insurance plan necessitated a transfer to a psychologist in private practice, whom she continued to see over the next year.

DISCUSSION

Rapport Building. Nora presented a different type of challenge in building rapport than most other clients in this volume: She had prior experience with psychotherapists and had terminated quickly with all of them. In part, this represented her fear of confronting the emotional aspect of her physical symptoms. She also

had high and unrealistic expectations for psychotherapy, especially for the speed of response to therapeutic intervention: She
wanted radical change in two or three sessions. I responded with
a dual message: I expressed confidence that therapy could be
helpful and also expressed certainty that it would not help in two
sessions. I also left the choice up to her, by describing what I
thought we would do initially in addressing her problems and
suggesting that it would be close to 6 months before we could
evaluate progress.

This approach created a very different situation from what she
had apparently experienced with other therapists. While expressing confidence that therapy would help, I did not encourage her
to decide in favor of it. I also directly addressed her ideas about
the length of time it should take and told her candidly that I could
not meet those expectations. As described above, she decided to
pursue therapy and delay evaluating results for a few months.
For those first several months, we would frequently confront her
impatience to have things change more quickly. The difference in
our perspectives on the time course of changing behavior and
emotional reactions became a standing joke between us. It was
helpful in this interaction that I saw her in a clinic where neither
the clinic nor I profited from prolonging the therapy.

Techniques in Therapy. If Nora had been able to use passive
relaxation techniques or exercise for relaxation, we would have
focused on these early on. Her health problems and general disposition ruled out exercise. Her history made it clear that passive
relaxation was equated with loss of control for her. For these reasons, we focused on self-monitoring and identifying causes of
stress, and then problem solving to eliminate stress where possible. In many cases, this led to changes in her approach to life,
often by eliminating activities that she had taken on somewhat
impulsively. In other instances, this approach led to relabeling as
enjoyable events that she had been considering stressful. For example, after trying for a few weeks to change her sleeping pattern,
she came to identify her time alone in the night and her afternoon
naps as pleasant parts of her life, rather than as signs of stress.

It also became apparent early in the therapy that Nora was almost entirely alexythymic (i.e., she had no ability to label her

emotions and talk about them). This lack of ability to identify and label emotion is emerging as a key problem that results in physical health problems as responses to stress (cf. Rodin & Salovey, 1989). Using focusing to identify the physical sensation component of emotions (Gendlin, 1978), and self-monitoring to identify when such sensations occurred outside of therapy, we were able to increase her ability to identify emotions and understand why they occurred when they occurred.

In her case, improvement in recognizing and talking about emotions as emotions was directly associated with decreasing complaints about physical distress. One example is the focusing on pain in her chest, which actually turned out to be discomfort in her throat, and then was identified as "I'm irritated and trying not to express it." Later, she came to identify formerly inexplicable waves of fatigue as extreme irritation, usually experienced in a group setting.

As she became more comfortable with her emotions and more competent in describing them, we began to talk about her family settings, both her family of origin and her current family. As is generally true, the prohibition against being emotional was traceable to rules learned in her family of origin, essentially equating emotionality with craziness and an unsuccessful life. Her husband was also experienced as a stern and stoic man who discouraged emotional expression.

The focus on the family called forth a richer range of emotional expression. There were numerous issues regarding feeling lonely and abandoned, even though she had moved away; feeling frustrated with her sister and her husband; and having felt that her family of origin had both pressured her to succeed and limited her in her attempts at success. She also had considerable, lifelong ambivalence about sex and her sexuality: She enjoyed sex but also found it shameful. She also had some regrets about having been so sheltered and shy during her young adult premarriage years. Never having had any sexual experience with other men, there was normal curiosity, which was clearly going to remain unsatisfied.

Being able to talk out and explore some of these issues and explore "what if" fantasies helped to set boundaries to her fears. Talking about her regrets about her sexual life made it clear that they were mild in degree and that she had no real desire to act out her fantasies. Exploring her irritations with her husband led to discussion of divorce and made it clear that she feared divorce much more than she resented her husband's imperfections.

Discussion of relationships with different family members tended to result in more open communication with them and setting limits on some relationships while accepting more responsibility for the state of others. For example, she came to realize and acknowledge that her daughters felt abandoned by her when she moved across the country from them. She also realized that she tended to cut one daughter off when she tried to talk to Nora about problems, because she suspected the daughter was doing things she would find hard to accept.

Gerontological Issues. Nora's focus on learning about emotionality calls attention to the differences in describing emotions that exist between age groups. As I have commented in describing working with Nora, I compromised on describing *anger* as *irritation*. I have found this a natural adaptation to working with older persons and feel that little is lost by this translation. I have also become aware, as I train new therapists to work with the elderly, that many young therapists become quite frustrated in working with an older client who is obviously experiencing anger, but argues with the younger therapist's use of this word for that emotion.

While I tend to think of this difference as due to differing socialization of earlier-born versus later-born cohorts, it is also possible that older adults really do not experience the same intensity of anger as do persons in young adulthood. Gynther (1979) argues that older adults are less prone to anger and impulsiveness. Schulz (1982) argues that emotionality in later life becomes more complex and less intensely experienced: Anger does not lend itself to complexity or subtlety. Less direct evidence from the cognitive coping literature (Felton & Revenson, 1987; Folkman, Lazarus, Pimley, & Novacek, 1987) suggests that older adults tend to use coping styles based on acceptance, rather than those based on confrontation. Certainly, there is no need to insist on using our words for the experience; perhaps there is reason to think we are projecting our younger view of the nature of the experience itself.

Nora is also representative of the manner in which a psychologically oriented approach to the older adult tends to move away from activity theory answers to the problems of late life. Nora was an avid believer in activities and a frequent volunteer; she also would find these activities both physically and emotionally overwhelming. Her devotion to being active was also, in general, an escape from other problems in her life, especially the family issues she wanted to avoid. Nora had to learn to limit the number of activities in which she involved herself and to be selective and choose activities that were helpful and enjoyable. To some extent, it was necessary to limit outside activity in order to improve relationships that were more personal: to be closer to her husband, to be more available to her daughters, and to have time to develop friendships. Following Botwinick (1984), it is these more personal connections, rather than formal activities, that relate to life satisfaction in later life (cf. Ward et al., 1984).

In a related vein, Nora's initial estrangement from her family is another common gerontological theme. The presumed isolation of the elderly has been a common theme in American popular culture and has remained so, even with evidence to the contrary (Shanas, 1979). Only occasionally is it suggested that the elderly may contribute to this isolation by their own personal characteristics (Bennet, 1983; Rook, 1984). In Nora's instance, we see a woman who moved away from family and felt abandoned by them. She also had to examine her interactive style in the family, and change aspects of it in order to be closer to them. While her family undoubtedly contributed to both the problem and the solving of it, we can learn from Nora that the elderly are not always passive victims of withdrawing family.

Relationship Issues. Nora was inclined to perceive me throughout much of the therapy as quiet, critical, and withholding. Since all of the description fit her perception of her husband, and only the first fits my usual style in therapy (based on self-perception and feedback from numerous clients), I felt there was some degree of transference of feelings for her husband to myself. In fact, she described her son-in-law and some male antagonists in groups in much the same terms, and there may have been a more general interference operating in her relationships with men.

As we started to focus more on her relationship with her husband, I was able to use these misperceptions of me as cues to

problems at home. I also began to challenge her perceptions of me
by describing what I was really thinking at times when she perceived me as either critical or thinking something I did not want
to tell her. In the former instances, I was often thinking something
quite positive about her and the progress she was making in therapy. In the latter, I was often trying to decide what I thought of
what she had just said, or trying to think what to do next, as opposed to having some wise thoughts or advice that I was withholding from her.

For myself, the therapy was complicated by the fact that Nora
reminded me of my mother. Although there were many differences, my mother had been very talkative and prone to somatic
complaints during much of my adolescent and early adult years.
Fortunately for myself and Nora, she was not the first person I
encountered who had these qualities, and I was readily aware of
the potential problem from the first session. Nonetheless, there
were moments when feelings more related to my mother than to
Nora would arise either in therapy or as I thought about her case.
In many instances, these would tend to leave me feeling pessimis-
tic about the outcome of therapy or helpless in confronting a
given problem, since I have never been especially effective in
helping my mother with what I believe to be her problems.

The more I have worked in psychotherapy with the elderly, the
more I feel that this type of error (parental countertransference) is
at the root of much pessimism with regard to working with older
adults. In talking about the elderly with students, other therapists, and journalists, I am constantly struck by how often examples are drawn from our own family lives and generalized to "older
people." While there are numerous logical problems with this approach to thinking about the elderly, it is perhaps most clear
when thinking about therapeutic pessimism. Few people have
much luck changing their parents' minds about issues of funda-
mental importance, especially issues on which parents and children
typically disagree. This observation says more about parent-child
relationships than about young-old relationships.

Certainly it has been my experience that older women clients
(most of whom are considerably older than my mother) are more
impressed with my clinical insights, whereas my mother remains

unconvinced by my opinions about how she should run her life. That's the way it is and the way it should be.

Summary. Nora presents an example of the interplay of emotional and physical problems in later life. In her life, many of her physical symptoms were caused by suppression of her emotions, failure to recognize the physical signs of emotion, and denial of conflict within the family. She also had physical symptoms that were caused by physical problems. With the older adult, it is both impossible and irresponsible to have a simplistic view of mind-body relationships. The coexistence of physical and emotional problems, the interactions between the two, and the possibility of either looking like the other must all be considered in working with the elderly.

CHAPTER THIRTEEN

Lana:
Psychosomatics and Overuse of Medical Services

Lana was in her early 60s when she initially sought out therapy because of feeling lonely and too fearful to go out for social activity. At the time we met, she had been divorced for more than 20 years after a long and unhappy marriage. Lana had been on disability for more than a decade, having worked for a few years in social service and paraprofessional counseling jobs after the divorce. Her disability had been granted for depression. She was now considered retired by virtue of her age.

She had been in psychotherapy most of those 20 years. In retrospect, she felt that the first and longest-term therapist had not helped her; whereas the second had been more goal-oriented and had encouraged her to terminate therapy after about 2 years. As might be expected with this background, she was excellent at playing the client role.

Her initial presentation of her problem was that she had moved to Ventura County out of Los Angeles about 18 months previously to escape from a destructive relationship with a long-term boyfriend. He was described as very bright and talented, but manic-depressive. They had been evicted from an apartment they were sharing, and he was in some trouble with the police for writing vaguely threatening letters to local government officials. Lana had moved in with her daughter, a single mother raising two children. Although Lana was vague about the details, her daughter had recently moved out to live with a boyfriend, leaving Lana with a place she could not afford. Lana fairly quickly found an apartment she could handle on her own.

She described feeling extremely isolated in Ventura. The people she met locally were not as bright or as interesting as people she had known in the city. When she tried to get out of her apartment, she often became highly anxious and panic-stricken. She saw herself as extremely frail physically as well. She had hypertension and mild heart problems and suffered from a little-known intestinal disorder, which had taken years to diagnose. During that time, she had often been labeled hypochondriacal.

She was also highly sensitive to medications, got side-effects easily, frequently had unusual allergic reactions, and almost always needed lower dosages than other people. Although she professed to have a low opinion of physicians and changed doctors often, her life centered around doctor visits. When we started therapy, she had an internist and two other specialists and was upset over not being able to get a referral to a third specialist.

My first strategy with Lana was to stay with a short-term, goal-oriented therapy. We agreed to work on her anxiety and on increasing her social activity. She had extensive exposure to various kinds of relaxation and meditation. After brief discussion, she agreed to start using one that had worked for her some years before. My role with this intervention was largely to monitor whether she was using it weekly, and to ask if she had thought of using her meditation when she described various anxiety-arousing situations.

Increasing her activity level proved more problematic. She had virtually no local social contacts. Her only regular interactions were with her daughter (almost always angry conversations that degenerated rapidly into threats), grandsons (usually involving requests for money or mutual complaining about their mother), and the "ex-boyfriend" who called frequently for long conversations and visited occasionally. Their relationship was also mostly argumentative, with recriminations about the past: who had left whom and who had let the other down most frequently. When asked why she maintained contact with him, her answer was that it was mostly sexual. Although her boyfriend was impotent due to his psychotropic medication, he enjoyed giving her pleasure.

In addition to these close relationships, Lana occasionally visited with a neighbor, whom she often found ignorant and offensive. Lana was an Italian former Catholic with an Anglo-Saxon last name from her ex-husband. The neighbor often made prejudiced remarks about various ethnic groups and Catholics.

Suggestions for groups and places she might try inevitably met with a "yes, but . . ." response. On the positive side, she had already researched the local senior social scene and the singles scene rather thoroughly; there was very little I could suggest that she did not already know about. On the other hand, she had tried many of them and found them lacking—often for good reasons that corresponded to reports from other, less characteristically negative clients. The ones she had not tried she had good reasons for not trying.

At the end of the weeks that it took to establish this picture, I suggested that we redefine her goals. In fact, she now stated that she had never had female friends and was not ready to start now. What she "really wanted" was a better boyfriend and better relationships with her family.

Discussing her family in some historical detail, the prospects were not encouraging. I asked when she and daughter had last gotten along well, and the answer was not since the daughter was about 14. She was now nearing 40. The daughter had been defiant and rebellious as a teenager, had left home as soon as she legally could, and had been distant and hostile ever since. It now developed that Lana had basically insisted on moving in with her daughter, over the daughter's objections, when she had left Los Angeles. While living together, Lana had disrupted one romantic relationship of the daughter's and had been involved in several disputes with her teenaged grandsons, who were not happy about losing a bedroom to her.

It was also revealed at this point that she had a son who lived in a neighboring state. There was little contact with him, due, she said, to his conversion to a Protestant church emphasizing strict morality. Her son now disapproved of her.

She also talked of a conflicted relationship with a sister in Northern California, who was alcoholic and very critical of Lana. In discussing the sister, it developed that Lana saw herself as the only nonalcoholic member of her family: Both parents had been heavy drinkers, and the children had been left to raise themselves and often to take care of their intoxicated parents. She never saw herself as part of this pattern, even though she had a history of rather heavy use of pain medications and tranquilizers. Her medications were, of course, all prescribed by physicians. She did at times acknowledge that she might have "an alcoholic personality."

Discussion of physical symptoms would often predominate for one third to one half of a session. These discourses would often be a nondiscriminated mixture of symptoms clearly related to her diagnosed physical ailments, physical symptoms rather clearly related to panic attacks, and less clearly defined symptoms. One of these, a tightness in her chest for which her physician could find no physical reason, led us to spend some time on the concept of emotions expressing themselves in physical terms when there was no other release.

A simplified focusing exercise rather quickly led to her identifying this feeling as suppressed anger and immediately relating it to her father having instructed her to never be angry. Lana was sufficiently therapy-trained and dramatic, so that we got more verbose expression of insight than was necessary. This session did become a turning point in therapy, however, in that she retained the ability to recognize this symptom as her expression of anger. She was able then to determine why she was angry and act on it in a fairly assertive way. She not only had been through assertion training but had also taught it in the past. While it took several months for her to *feel* angry more directly, this insight was the basis of her first lasting change in therapy and underlined the role of emotions in her physical health: realms that she had previously kept quite separate.

Unfortunately, soon after this, Lana fell while leaving a local store, which left her with mild back pain and increased emotional distress. She became involved for several months with more physicians, a chiropractor, an acupressure therapist, an attorney, and another psychologist. She often missed appointments. The ones she kept were mostly taken up discussing her "case," and my unwillingness to write a report saying she was more depressed after the accident. I had, in fact, never seen her feeling so good emotionally. We also discussed my concern about her having two therapists at once. I insisted that she choose one of us in order to keep the therapy focused. To my surprise, she did, and chose me.

As the busy-ness of the case subsided, Lana seemed to become more serious about and more focused on the work of therapy. She now only rarely spoke in terms of physical symptoms, but began to explore her life history in search of the emotions that she had suppressed for years. She was genuinely surprised to discover herself as an angry woman: Her self-image had been that of a passive, sensitive victim of fate. Her anger constantly brought up images of her childhood.

She had taken care of her parents, but had been ignored by them. Her father had been on disability for years while her mother worked, complained, and drank. Lana would come home from school and do the cooking and sometimes put him to bed. She had apparently been able to suppress her disappointment and anger for 50 years, while also learning from her father that being disabled was a way to get special treatment from others.

Her marriage and child-raising years were largely blank in her historical memory. She now saw her former husband as boring. She was upset about not really discovering sexual satisfaction until after their divorce. It was only after the divorce that she worked and rather quickly found a way to collect disability pay. She had somewhat vague memories of bland happiness when her children were small. She found their adolescence intolerable. Since they had become adults, her interactions seemed to focus on trying to get them to take care of her and on her disappointment that they did not. A number of specific examples showed that while she wanted advice and consolation from her daughter, she deeply resented and often hostilely rejected her daughter's calls for advice or support.

After exploring this history and acknowledging her anger, Lana lapsed into depression and a deeply felt sense of loneliness. This state was deepened in that she had also very gradually tapered off the relationship with her former boyfriend. It had become clear, over a period of several months, that her most severe periods of emotional turmoil were connected to his visits and to their lengthy phone calls. She had reached the decision in a slow and ambivalent manner. At one point, she came in and announced that he was moving up and they were getting married. However, she had decided to end it and was eventually able to do so.

Although addressed in therapy only as an example of her self-defeating struggles with authority, Lana significantly changed her relationship to physicians during therapy. She became less critical and abusive of her doctors, reduced the number she was seeing, and gradually reduced her visits to them. She had come to see physicians as being there to help with physical problems, rather than as sources of comfort and consolation or as substitute fathers with whom she could be angry for not caring enough. In fact, she went so far in reinterpreting physical symptoms that she had to be strongly encouraged to seek help for a serious skin rash, which she was interpreting as stemming from anxiety. Her physician diagnosed it as an allergic reaction to some medication she was taking.

At this point, she was less anxious; she was spending less of her time in doctor's offices; she had a better relationship with her doctor; she had more intellectual understanding of her self-defeating interactions with others; and she was quite depressed and lonely. She remained largely unwilling either to explore options for social activity or try to make new friends.

In this later phase of my therapy with her, she moved into a group-therapy setting. Her social problems were thrown into clear relief within this group, in that she rarely even acknowledged other people's problems and clearly wanted only to tell her own. She was generally critical of whatever advice she was given. At one point she literally minimized another member's struggle with terminal illness as less significant than her own psychosomatic pains, because the other woman's problem wouldn't last as long and she knew what the cause was. Her interaction with her daughter stood out as especially self-centered and nonreciprocal within a group that was characterized by problem-ridden and distant parent-child relationships. She did make some moves to go out to museums and special exhibits locally and was developing a relationship with a female friend when I left the clinic.

DISCUSSION

Rapport Building. My first contact with Lana was a telephone call to my private practice office. In this initial contact, she gave a lengthy description of her problems and made several special requests: She wanted to be seen more than once a week; she wanted to know if I could refer her for medication; and she needed reduced fees. The total picture was sufficiently complex that I immediately decided to refer her to the multidisciplinary team, where I had better resources and she could have a reduced fee.

While Lana seemed to have no problem forming a dependent attachment to me as the therapist, I had some difficulty from the beginning feeling connected to her as a client. While there were practical issues as well, the core reaction was simply that I did not like her very much. She talked a great deal and had mastered therapeutic jargon and concepts. She complained about physical symptoms, and she was bitter and somewhat hostile toward others while professing a great and immediate attachment to me. On the more professional, task-oriented side, I saw her as a challenging and interesting client who was likely to be very difficult. I felt certain that she would stretch my therapeutic skills and that I would be able to help her, if she stayed with the therapy. I doubted from the beginning that she would.

In general, my personal experience as a therapist has been that personal liking for clients is not very closely associated with success in the sense of the client's achievement of therapeutic goals. I have had clients whom I disliked, or who were quite difficult for me, who made excellent progress—and clients whom I liked very much who did not change at all.

I found myself liking Lana several months into the therapy. The combination of her insight into the role of emotion in her physical symptoms, along with my greater understanding of why she did some of the things she did as we explored her life history together, made her a more comprehensible and likable person in my eyes. This change in basic feeling for her did not blind me to her continuing problems in relating to others in her life and her almost complete inability to comprehend that other people had problems also.

Techniques in Therapy. As has been my tendency throughout my career as a therapist, I started therapy with Lana by focusing on her initial presenting problems in a goal-oriented focused manner. Recognizing her long involvement in therapy, I also used her previous experience to guide what we needed to do first. In these first sessions, much of the work was in identifying problems and then asking what she had done in the past that would help.

This approach helped her in three ways: (a) to straighten out her housing problem, which she had more information and skills to deal with than did I; (b) to identify a helpful relaxation method; and (c) to start working on increased social activity, mostly by identifying what did not work and what she did not want to try.

The next phase of her therapy consisted largely of working on translating some of her physical symptoms into emotions and talking about her relationship with her physicians. I led her through a process of identifying which symptoms and sensations she thought were due to illnesses she had, which were due to medications, and which were thought to be unexplainable by all of the doctors she had seen. I then explained that emotions can make symptoms worse or can be perceived as physical sensations. While doing this, I emphasized that emotion-induced symptoms hurt just as much and are just as real as those with clear biomedical causes. With this background she was able to recognize the emotional relevance of some symptoms, so much so that she had to be cautioned to seek physical assessment of some new symptoms that appeared.

Throughout this period she continued to argue with physicians, feel misunderstood by them, change physicians in response to these problems, and then get angry again when the new ones confirmed what the former ones had said. My role was to listen, note patterns and consistencies in her role and their advice, and gradually begin to question whether she was getting anywhere by ignoring their advice and constantly switching to new doctors. With a lot of repetition in a calm and nonconfrontive manner, she began to hear the regularities herself. I gradually introduced some humor about the pattern, which enabled her to distance herself from it and begin to criticize what she was doing and examine her expectations of the physicians.

Clinically it is of interest in understanding the role of life review in therapy to note that Lana is the only person in this volume whose life review is not connected to grieving or to accepting one's own death. In her case, the review served more to reinterpret her life in light of the new concept that she had unexpressed emotions, as opposed to perceiving herself as suffering from many mysterious physical problems. This new concept led to understanding many past events differently and to seeing new relationships between her past and the present. One practical consequence was a striking change in her attitude and behavior toward physicians.

This phase also led into much discussion of her relationships with family members: parents, her sister, her children (we spent some time discussing a son that she had never mentioned before), and her grandchildren. While she seemed to gain some conceptual insight from these talks, it appears to me that none of her family relationships changed as a result. The only person I met from among her significant others was the ex-boyfriend, and therapy seemed to lead to her putting more limits on his demands and then to terminating that relationship.

I had hopes that group therapy would assist her in gaining new interpersonal skills, but during the time we were working in group together, there was no evidence that this happened. If anything, her actions in group served to give me a new perspective on how completely unperceptive she was about others and on the very high level of nonreciprocal demands that she placed on family. With regard to desire for social contact and new friends, Lana seemed to be more willing to lower her expectations and remain lonely than to change in ways that would bring her close to others.

Gerontological Issues. Lana obviously illustrates points about the role of health psychology issues in counseling the elderly that have already been made in earlier chapters. While some writers have viewed the tendency toward talking about physical symptoms as a distracting behavior of older adults that must be corrected, I tend on the whole to see such talk as a normal part of later life in most cases, and in cases like Lana's, as a valid focus for therapy. The literature on personality and aging has tended to confirm that the increased talk about physical symptoms is related to common physical changes in later life, rather than increased hypochondriasis (Costa & McCrae, 1985).

While older people can and do use physical symptoms to avoid talking about emotional issues, in most instances the therapist's discomfort with physically oriented talk is best seen as an issue with which the therapist needs assistance. Many young adults, and especially those with a psychological worldview, are made profoundly uncomfortable by the evidence of physical limitation that is a daily experience of many older people.

Lana's story speaks most strongly to the twin issues of the persistence of problems throughout the life span that are rooted in the family of origin, especially when that family is violent or otherwise severely dysfunctional. Lana's particular experiences led to a lifetime of substance misuse, to use of the sick role as a means both to earn money and elicit caring from others, and to serious and persistent disturbance in her ability to form connection with others.

Probably because such issues have only relatively recently become the focus of media attention and public discussion, there seems to be a tendency to overlook themes of child abuse, molestation, incest, abortion, and rape in the lives of older adults. Both client report and history argue that none of these are recent inventions, although it is clearly more acceptable to talk about them now than in past decades. Such themes rather commonly occur in the early histories of older adults seeking psychotherapy for psychological distress, even when the distress appears to be acute and occurring for the first time in late life.

The question of how much change can be expected, when the problem is of such long standing, is a major theme in the literature on psychotherapy with the elderly and is of relevance for our understanding of personality throughout the life span. Karl Abraham's (1919/1977) dictum, that it is the age of the neurosis rather than the age of the client that predicts success, still points to pessimism about change of such characterological traits in the older client. Rechtschaffen's (1959) review of literature on psychotherapy with the elderly reports the generally optimistic view of those working with older clients, and even includes the warning that the elderly may be overly susceptible to change. I have tended to side with the latter viewpoint.

Coming from a background in cognitive behavioral/social learning theory, my general view is that behavior is determined at least as much by environmental contingencies as by enduring traits that are stronger than the person who has them. It further seems to me that the lives of older adults are in many ways less restricted by the work and family expectations that inhibit change in younger adults (Knight, 1986).

Lana provides an instructive example. She changed her relationship to her own emotions and reconstructed her view of

herself and her life history in her late 60s. This resulted in major
changes in the way she spent her life, including ending a dysfunctional love relationship and beginning to explore friendship with
women for the first time in her life.

On the other hand, there were clearly areas in which change
was anything from limited to nonexistent. I have no way of knowing whether the lack of progress in relationship with family was
due to her unwillingness to change in this area, or to the other
members of her family system persisting in their patterns even as
she attempted to change. Certainly, Lana was still captive to the
unresolved problems of her family of origin as she raised her children, and they still actively resented their upbringing even as
they raised their own children.

There was also some sense of unwillingness to change, or at
least unwillingness to work as hard as would be necessary to
make new friends. I have commented on this decision in earlier
chapters as a frequent outcome of discussing new friendships late
in life. In Lana's case, it also reminds me of the common psychotherapy dictum (I have heard it attributed to Fritz Perls, Harry
Stack Sullivan, and others) that "people want to feel better but
they don't want to change." In short, it seems to me that older
clients have the same right as young ones to decide not to achieve
therapeutic goals. Hopefully, they will also have access to therapists who have not decided a priori that older adults cannot
change lifelong patterns.

Relationship Issues. The principal transferential issue in the
therapeutic relationship with Lana was an erotic one. Lana was
seductive in a variety of ways throughout much of our relationship. On our first meeting, she was gushy about the sense of closeness she had felt while talking with me on the telephone. Much of
her interaction with me had mildly suggestive overtones. She
would often bring up stories about older women having sexual
relationships with younger men. There were also stories about
younger men being attracted to her. The point in the therapy at
which she was seeing another psychologist related to her disability claims felt very much like being involved in a love triangle.
She seemed to enjoy both the illicit nature of the other contact and

setting up a situation in which I would force her to choose between us.

Most of the time, this transference was a background to the therapy and served mostly to cement the connection between us. I never confronted her directly on this issue, feeling that to do so would be a message that she was no longer desirable. I did, in fact, consent to her requests for hugs at the end of sessions as a way of reaffirming her femininity. At the same time, I never saw her outside the office, nor in the office when I was the only one there. The hugs were on the way out of the office, where the receptionist could see what happened.

I used my awareness of the mildly erotic nature of her feelings to guide me through planning an overall course of the relationship that would be different from what she had experienced before. I was consistently available and honest, but also unmanipulatable and able to set limits (e.g., on number and length of phone calls between sessions).

As an example, my refusal to write a letter in support of her increased disability after her fall was a test of her ability to manipulate me. I was candid with her about my impression of her improvement in mood and firm about my unwillingness to do something that I considered unethical. I also pointed out that she retained control of the overall situation, in that she owned the confidentiality of our visits and I could not testify against her without her express permission. This incident is likely the first time that she experienced disagreeing with someone she was close to without angry words on either side. I was still surprised when she decided to continue the therapy with me.

On my side, I think the major countertransferential issue was my reaction to her high level of dependency needs. This reaction undoubtedly accounts for some of my initial dislike of her. Having the experience of managing her dependency and not feeling overwhelmed by her needs likely accounts for my increasing comfort with her as the therapy went on. It has doubtless been helpful to me in other areas of my life, including preparing me for fatherhood.

Summary. Lana presents another example of physical symptoms being rooted in unacknowledged emotion. In her case, this problem is complicated by long-term deficits in relating to others, which grew out of her dysfunctional family of origin. These relational deficits, combined with the expression of emotion in physical symptom equivalents, led to a long series of disturbed relationships with physicians. These relationships were self-defeating for her and undoubtedly extremely unpleasant for the physicians, who probably wondered justifiably what they had done to deserve such treatment. The psychotherapist can often do much to improve the client's relationship to the physician by helping the client to understand what she or he is hoping for and what can reasonably be expected.

CHAPTER FOURTEEN

Lila and Sophia:
Paranoid Psychosis in Late Life

Among the more severe mental disorders of late life, paranoid symptoms seem to be more salient than in the psychoses of young adulthood (cf. Roth, 1987, for an historical review). Contrary to popular thinking, but consistent with nearly a century of expert observation, late onset psychosis is often more benign than early onset disorders and there is evidence that early onset schizophrenia often improves with age (Miller & Cohen, 1987). In this chapter, the two older women presented appear to have developed paranoid psychoses with first onset late in life.

LILA

Lila was brought in for a consultation by her niece, who was concerned that Lila was becoming senile. She had been complaining about prowlers and for the past few weeks had refused to eat the meals brought by the local Meals on Wheels program because she thought the food was being tampered with. Lila had been widowed for several decades and had no children. Her niece, who was more than 60, was her closest relative and main social support. The niece was quite distressed and anxious about Lila's condition.

Lila was older than 70 and very well groomed. She spoke excellent, although deliberate and accented English. Of White Russian background, she had left Russia in 1917 and had lived in China until the 1940s, when she emigrated to California. She was direct about her problem, which she presented as being harassed by youngsters in the neighborhood who ran through her backyard and upset her trash cans at night. She also thought that the house had been entered and things had been stolen, but these concerns were more vague. She could not describe what was missing.

She explained the discrepancy between her view of the problem and her niece's by stating that her niece was "a very nervous girl" and could not believe that there could be problems in Lila's neighborhood because it was in a decent part of town. Lila argued that even kids from decent neighborhoods enjoy harassing old ladies with foreign accents. With regard to the food, she denied having said it was tampered with, but said she had noticed a change in quality a few weeks earlier and thought maybe they had a new cook who had not learned her job yet.

She agreed to take, and did very well on, mental status testing to screen for memory impairment. She denied any problems with depression or anxiety, other than being worried about what these kids would do next. The police had been called, but no one was there when the officers arrived and they were impatient with her stories. Her concerns were interfering with her sleep, and she had lost a few pounds lately but was still moderately overweight. She felt the food would improve soon and agreed to eat more in order to appease her niece.

At the end of this first interview, I was quite perplexed. The niece had presented a number of concerns that sounded like dementing illness or psychosis. There was no evidence of dementia, and the suspicions that Lila voiced were solidly within the "gray zone" of being like paranoid delusions but also quite plausible and possibly solidly based in reality. It also appeared to me that the niece was considerably more anxious than Lila was. In the last few minutes, I decided to "fish" for more distorted thinking and simply asked Lila whether she had experienced any other unusual or disturbing events in the past few weeks.

She paused and looked at me for several seconds and then stated matter-of-factly that the birds on the tree outside her kitchen window were bothering her. I asked what they were doing and she said that they spoke to her and said "terrible things." When I asked what sort of things they said, Lila blushed and told me that she could not repeat them to me, but they were very insulting and embarrassing and that "an old woman should not have to put up with such language and insults."

In our next interview, we talked more about the birds and what they were saying and doing. Interestingly, once she was able to discuss the birds, her complaints about the food and the neighborhood kids decreased rapidly to zero. I introduced the idea that our psychiatrist might be able to give her medicine that would help her sleep and calm her nerves. She acknowledged that her nerves were very upset by these foul-mouthed birds.

Over a period of four sessions or so, she eventually agreed to see our psychiatrist. She had some anxiety about the medication but more reluctance to being treated by a female doctor. She had more confidence in me (at the time, a barely 30-year-old male) than in our 50ish female psychiatrist.

We also scheduled a family session with Lila, the niece, and a grandniece who was home from college. They were highly anxious about Lila and concerned that they needed to do something: basically, move her to a retirement home. After a general discussion of the issues, they agreed to wait and see what counseling and medication would do for Lila, who not only agreed to eat regularly but also pointed out that she had not called the police in several weeks. After some rather pointed comments from Lila, the other two also acknowledged that they were "always worried," and if it was not Lila, they would be worrying about something or someone else. In fact, they were both highly anxious women.

As the medication took effect over the next few weeks, the birds' commentary shifted from obnoxious and obscene to pleasantly irrelevant. With this change, there was less need for our sessions, so she shifted over to monthly visits with the psychiatrist. A few years later, increasing physical frailty led to her moving to a residential care facility. She later passed away without any recurrence of her psychotic thinking.

SOPHIA

I first met Sophia after her release from the state psychiatric hospital in our area. A close friend and colleague, who was working on the geropsychiatric unit there, had called and arranged for me to follow up on Sophia's mental health care after release to a residential care facility. She had described Sophia as verbal, intelligent, and charming, though acutely paranoid. In the previous year, she had been kicked out of three residential care facilities for hostility or bizarre behavior and had been admitted to the county inpatient psychiatric unit each time and to the state hospital twice. It was felt that she had finally been stabilized on antipsychotic medication during this last hospitalization, which had lasted several months. The referring colleague, a social work intern, had felt that Sophia had established a relationship with her and that this contact was an important part of the new stability.

Sophia was older than 70 and a cultured, well groomed, Polish-American woman. She moved and spoke with great dignity. She was well educated for her cohort, with some postsecondary education. She had been married to a professional man, and her son was an engineer who was doing well. Her husband had died more than 10 years earlier, and she described a normal, if difficult grieving process. She had found widowhood boring and had done some housework for people in Beverly Hills and Bel Air. After an ill-defined dispute with her last employer, she had moved to Chicago and lived in the Polish community there for several years, returning to California about 3 years prior to our first contact. She had not done well since her return.

There were disputes with landlords and neighbors, then moving into residential care and a number of arguments and fights there. Most of these disputes involved her confronting people whom she knew were conspiring to kill her or kidnap her, or were poisoning her food. She was anti-Semitic and also still quite fearful of Nazis. Her delusions centered on plots by Jews, the FBI, and the Gestapo.

She was quite intelligent and did very well on mental status questions. Her English was not good. Her son stated that she had been much more fluent prior to her move to Chicago, where she had lived in the Polish neighborhood for 7 years and had spoken no English.

Since she had been primed by her counselor at the hospital for our relationship, she virtually instantly formed a strong attachment for me. She was impressed by my specializing in working with older people and by my educational background. She had also decided, after the multiple hospitalizations, that she needed to take her "nerve medication."

Her conversations were often quite normal and free from distortion. We discussed her problems in adjusting to the residential care home in which she lived. She had some normal disagreements and conflicts with other residents. She felt a sense of loss over her declining social status. We discussed in some detail her past in Poland and in Southern California while her husband was still alive. She was surprised, hurt, and saddened to find herself a psychiatric patient living in residential care homes. She was very upset that most of the other residents and the home's owners were not her intellectual equals. While this clearly had a paranoid flavor, it was also objectively accurate.

She was always more candid with me than with the psychiatrist about her delusions. With her permission, I would accompany her into the psychiatrist's office and describe her increasing nervousness as she got into conflicts with the home's residents or owners. She frequently began to wonder if the owners had connections to the Gestapo. At one point she became convinced that they were operating a house of prostitution with the other female residents (all older than 75 and either demented or chronically mentally ill) as the "girls." Changes in medication generally reduced these concerns within the week. We continued to meet once or twice a month.

She drew a great sense of security from our visits and from our relationship. After the first year, our program relocated to a different building, where I had a spacious office. On her first visit, she looked around and stated, "You're too young to have an office like this," and laughed. She tended to view me as a powerful and protective person. Gradually, she came to accept my advice which was often about the reality of some of her fears or her feelings that she was in any immediate danger. When she was becoming more delusional, her comfort was often simply in the equally delusional conviction that I was a powerful and protective authority who could hold the FBI at bay.

Unfortunately, after a couple of years, she became acutely agitated one evening and insisted on searching the owners of her residential care facility for concealed weapons. She was readmitted to the county psychiatric unit and quickly stabilized on

medications. The facility owners refused to take her back, so she
was placed in another home, where she stayed for the next several
years.

Over the last few years that I knew Sophia, her English gradually worsened and she spoke in Polish more and more often. She
also got lost walking in the neighborhood of the retirement home
and began to forget aspects of her past. This was interpreted as
the onset of a dementing illness, in addition to the paranoia that
she had displayed for more than 10 years without cognitive impairment. Finally, she seldom spoke in English and seemed to
have little recall of our visits or for who I was, so our relationship
ended.

DISCUSSION

Rapport Building. Since the essential nature of paranoid disorders is distrust of others, clearly building rapport with paranoid
clients and potential clients is quite difficult. After several mistakes in this area, I devoted considerable effort to learning how to
best approach paranoid clients. My beginning place was the excellent and practical chapter by MacKinnon and Michaels (1971).
Following their advice, I have developed a more formal style with
paranoid clients. This style tends to emphasize my role and status
as a professional and offers my availability to the clients, without
pushing myself on them or appearing to care very much if they
accept my offer to assist them. This style is quite different from my
approach with depressed and anxious clients, who tend to re-
spond to a more informal and more caring presentation by the
therapist.

I have, in general, made it a point to be scrupulously honest with
paranoid individuals and to try to avoid discussing my thoughts
about their delusions until the relationship is strongly established. Thus, while I listen carefully, I neither confirm nor deny
the reality of their suspicions in the first several sessions of clinical contact.

In my first contacts with older paranoid adults while doing outreach work, I focus only on getting to know them and getting
their permission for the next visit. I try to emphasize the control

that the potential client has over deciding about future visits. When that control is complete, I verbalize that explicitly. If there are limits, I state what those limits are. For example, if my visits are delaying an eviction action or a hospitalization, I tell the client that directly, so that he or she can make an informed decision.

I have noted that one of the most common mistakes that others make is in trying to accomplish too much too quickly. This rapid approach will, of course, evoke a refusal to cooperate, which tends to confirm the helper's pessimism about working with paranoid people. My approach tends more toward the salesman's maxim that you do not ask customers any questions to which they will say "no." With appropriate pacing, I have often been able to have a paranoid client, who was very angry about my first visit, sign up for therapy and agree to medication by the fourth or fifth contact.

I feel that medication is generally of great importance in the treatment of paranoid states and is, in fact, the treatment of choice; however, it has often been my experience that some psychosocial counseling is necessary to get the client to the point of consenting to take medication. This is particularly true of the late onset paranoid client, or of persons who have avoided mental health treatment for years. This experience with the interrelationship of psychosocial and medical interventions with psychotic elderly is similar to that described by Gene Cohen (1987).

The two older women described here represent two levels of late onset paranoia. One was living in the community, with relatively few problems; the other had an extensive history of psychiatric hospitalization and sheltered living arrangements. Both were somewhat atypically receptive to establishing an ongoing relationship with me. However, both exemplify the principles described here for establishing rapport: My relationship was more formal, with more emphasis on my status as a professional. I was direct and available, but not friendly or supportive in the same manner as with other clients described in this book. Finally, while I have progressed with other clients to a level of providing reality testing for some of their delusions, I never challenged the delusions of these two clients, but simply acknowledged the emotional reaction they were having to life as they perceived it.

Techniques in Therapy. In the majority of my work with older paranoid clients, the bulk of the work has consisted of establishing and maintaining the relationship. Once the relationship is established, setting up or encouraging the continuation of psychotropic medication is generally an essential part of treatment. I have generally found that adherence to medication is a continual issue, and that virtually any stressor will cause the clients to reconsider the medication and their relationship with the treating psychiatrist. It is, of course, quite easy for medication to become the focus of delusions about persecution and being poisoned.

In some particular cases, it is possible to go further in therapeutic work, and I have tended to follow a stress reduction model in those instances. In this model, the therapy focuses on teaching the client to recognize sources of stress that are associated with increased feeling of being persecuted. Once listed, it is often possible to find ways to reduce the total amount of stress and/or to avoid certain stressful situations. The major difference in pursuing this kind of counseling with very paranoid individuals, in terms of the content and techniques of therapy, is that the types of stressors are often different and minor, as compared with stressors that upset nonpsychotic clients. That is, while anyone would be stressed by being evicted from an apartment, a paranoid client may be nearly equally stressed by unexpectedly passing her landlord on the street.

My within-session conversation is governed by learning principles, as applied to my responses to the client's verbal behavior. I work toward reinforcing their accurate perceptions and their self-esteem and their sense of control over life, while putting their unrealistic thoughts on an extinction schedule (neither reinforced nor punished, but blandly disregarded). This interaction tends to increase the proportion of time spent in reality-based conversation. I do, however, encourage clients who need to share their delusions to talk with me about them, rather than with friends and family who are upset by such talk.

Gerontological Issues. Perhaps the major gerontological issue brought up by these two cases is the simple fact of the existence of the severely mentally ill older adult. Relatively little has been written about the psychotic elderly, even though schizophrenics grow old, and late onset paranoia has been recognized for years. For the person working in aging services, these older adults are often seen as depressed, eccentric, or demented, unless and until their delusions emerge as the relationship gets closer, or there is a recurrence of an acute episode.

The failure to recognize this group of older adults is both more curious and more tragic, given that the history of deinstitutionalization in mental health has left many of the chronic mentally ill elderly in HUD housing for the elderly, in downtown single-room-occupancy hotels, and in residential care facilities for the elderly (cf. Carl Cohen, 1987). From these settings, they become frequent visitors in senior recreation centers, senior meal sites, and some adult day-care settings.

When properly understood, the psychotic older adult can be integrated into such settings with few problems and can often be an especially helpful and insightful participant. However, if too many demands are made for closeness in relationships, participation in groups, or confrontation of fears that appear irrational to others, delusions and bizarre behavior are likely to emerge and frighten other participants and the staff as well. As noted by Gene Cohen (1987), much of consultative intervention in such settings can be understood as increasing the staff's understanding of psychosis and reducing their expectations for the psychotic older service user.

An indirect lesson from working with paranoid older adults is that many of the same skills used to establish rapport with these irrationally suspicious elderly persons are also useful with another group of distrustful older adults: the abused elderly. The same pattern of going slow, concentrating on building a relationship, and simply trying to maintain contact at first, described in the "Rapport Building" section here, is also useful with abused elderly. All too often the abuse report creates a sense of crisis and a felt need on the helper's part to do something immediately. If the victim is in physical danger, emergency action may be necessary. Otherwise, any attempt to intervene quickly is likely to be perceived by the victim as threatening and abusive, regardless of the intentions of the helping professional.

Relationship Issues. Both of the women described in this chapter established relationships with me that emphasized my status, power, and protective ability to a transferential degree. Especially with Sophia, there were times when I clearly became incorporated in her delusional world as a positive and protective figure who could keep her safe from those who were conspiring to kill her. These psychotic images of me were reduced, along with other delusions, as stressors decreased or medication was increased. Otherwise, these generally positive transferences were helpful to treatment and not bothersome to the clients.

Responding to such relationships can be distressing for the therapist. Especially with Sophia, whom I saw early in my career, I was initially somewhat uncomfortable with being seen as such an authority figure. I have since encountered similar discomfort in other therapists-in-training, who are often inclined to discount the power of their role in order to minimize their importance to the client, or in response to the therapist's motivated low self-esteem. Understanding the importance of being seen as a powerful authority figure as part of helping certain types of clients is a useful lesson for the therapist. It is also a lesson that can lead to an appropriate understanding of the power of the therapeutic role: one that leads neither to minimizing that power, so that mistakes can be ignored, nor to potential abuse of that power with passive and dependent clients.

My relationship with Lila was relatively brief and free from distortions on my part. I saw Sophia over a period of several years. After the first 2 years, the visits were less frequent and often brief. I became sufficiently attached to her, however, that I had considerable difficulty in recognizing her increasing cognitive impairment. It was only when she was no longer able to converse in even a limited manner in English that I gave up visiting. In retrospect, I suspect that during the last year or more of visits (probably about 10 actual contacts) she was able to recognize me only as a familiar person and had very little comprehension of what I said. The experience of making this mistake taught me much about the way in which a sense of emotional connection to a dementing person can obscure disability, that is readily apparent to others, and can lead to bad decisions about the need for continued treatment.

In what I take to be similar situations, I have seen case workers fight to keep people in their homes who were obviously not doing well at home, and have also seen residential care owners cited for license violations because they could not send a particularly beloved resident to a skilled nursing facility. While not justifying the errors, I can sympathize with the emotions that lead to such mistakes.

Summary. Working with the paranoid elderly requires not only special skills in building relationships with very distressed people but also the ability to tolerate working within their clearly delusional worldviews. A better understanding of them is important for mental health specialists and also for people who work with the elderly in general. Historically, both the aging network and the mental health system have tended to ignore the existence of the older schizophrenic. They sometimes appear for services anyway, and if they are incorrectly understood, the services they receive are likely to worsen rather than improve their condition.

CHAPTER FIFTEEN

Mildred:
Living on the Margins of Society

I first met Mildred while running a satellite outreach office in a Housing Authority apartment building on the lower-income side of town. She came in to see me in some distress and very concerned that she would be labeled as "crazy" and put away. Her concern was somewhat vague in focus, but she felt that one of her current caseworkers for an aging support services program did not like her very much and might try to have her institutionalized because of her mental health treatment background.

In fact, Mildred had spent a number of years of her life in mental health treatment. She had been in and out of state psychiatric hospitals throughout her adult life. The episodes of treatment had lasted anywhere from weeks to years. Her recollection was that she had usually been diagnosed as suffering for depression, but had also been labeled several times as having schizophrenia and once as being retarded.

At the time that I met her, she had not been in the state facility in more than 10 years and had been hospitalized once or twice during that time for a few days each in the county psychiatric ward. She had lived in various board-and-care homes and had follow-up psychiatric care for medication, as well as follow-up casework through a special program for persons released from psychiatric inpatient hospitals. At this time, she was not on medication and was living in a HUD-subsidized apartment with in-home supportive services and had caseworkers in both of those programs.

In our interview, Mildred appeared anxious to a high degree. Her speech was somewhat fast and she jumped from topic to topic. She was mildly agitated, twisting her fingers and squirming in the chair. She complained of panic attacks in which her heart pounded and she became short of breath. She was very verbal and appeared quite bright. Mildred gave a fairly well organized presentation of her case history. She felt that she had had problems with depression in the past. She had threatened suicide several times over the years and had made a few attempts by overdose. By her own description, these were always either situations where she would be found soon or times when she took pills and then called the ambulance herself. She denied delusions and hallucinations now or ever in her history.

Since much of her panic centered on the likelihood of being committed again, she asked for and was given psychological testing. Her MMPI profile showed a high level of distress on most of the clinical scales, but was a profile associated with intense distress and "identity crisis" types of reactions rather than psychosis. A review of available information from her history in the mental health department revealed that her last admissions were based on crises and were very short term, and she was given diagnoses suggestive of situational distress. Her case record had allusions to depressive and schizoaffective diagnoses, the latter apparently based primarily on her prior hospitalization record.

A call to the state hospital, with her permission, revealed only that her last admission was so long ago that the records were no longer available. Based on this evidence and my impressions from the clinical interview, I started therapy with her on the assumption that she was currently a highly anxious older woman with an unusual and dysfunctional history.

Much of this early phase of working with Mildred consisted of reassuring her about her own mental state. She was quite impressed with the results of the testing, which showed that she was not "crazy," and it proved very helpful for her to rethink her emotional state as being in an acute crisis but still in touch with reality. This realization in itself lowered her anxiety level considerably.

Her next concern was over the likelihood of being readmitted to the state hospital. I reassured her that this was considerably more difficult in the present than it had been at the time of her last admission. I further explained how such decisions got made and that, unless the circumstances were extreme, I, as her therapist, would effectively have veto power over an attempt to admit her. Again, this information was highly reassuring for her.

In this context, we discussed her prior admissions to state hospitals. She had been admitted once by her father when she was a young woman. She professed to have no idea why this admission had taken place. One of her husbands (she had been married and divorced four times, no children) had dropped her off at the hospital as they were breaking up after a stormy relationship. She had been admitted once after an overdose. Her more recent admissions for short stays had generally involved arguments with people where she was staying. Although always charming with me, she clearly had a tendency to get into disagreements with other people, which accelerated rapidly into agitated confrontations. She had, however, never hit anyone nor been hit during one of these arguments.

During these same early sessions, we discussed her problems with the caseworker in some detail and discovered some basis for the conflict. They had several practical difficulties over the number of hours of in-home care that Mildred was supposed to receive and over Mildred's complaints about various housekeepers who had been assigned under the program. In brief, Mildred wanted these women to put in the hours they were paid for and to do a job that met her standards. The caseworker's stance, as reported by Mildred, was that she did not really need as many hours as she had been given and that she should be grateful for the work that got done, not critical of what was not done. When Mildred persisted, the arguments would heat up and the caseworker would bring up Mildred's mental health history. This, of course, would anger and frighten Mildred even more.

We went through some role play and assertion training on this issue. Mildred was quite good at both of these, having had extensive classes and group work in the hospitals and in day-treatment programs. The major changes in her interaction with the caseworker were to add more positive comments about the worker and the program, and to be careful not to become overly anxious during these talks by reminding herself that the worker actually had very little power over her. In fact, as we discussed and rehearsed these discussions, Mildred spontaneously acknowledged that she did not need all the hours she had been assigned, and volunteered to relinquish some of them. This action either pleased or startled the caseworker so much that she became quite friendly toward Mildred.

With the immediate crisis resolved, Mildred then became quite depressed. She was acutely aware of being labeled as an old woman and as a mental patient. I was surprised by the latter because, unlike some other older people with long histories of psychiatric treatment, she had nothing in her appearance or mannerisms to suggest long term mental illness. She revealed to me that she often volunteered the information to people as she got to know them, sometimes in initial conversations. She would then be insulted or hurt either by the remarks people made or by their withdrawal.

I suggested that there was really no point in bringing up her history. After discussing the injustice and the inaccuracy of the stigma at some length, she acknowledged that it was unlikely that she would change anyone's mind and that her goal was improved contacts with people. She reduced the frequency of her self-disclosure, and her daily interactions with people improved rather dramatically over the next several months.

Her struggle with age stereotypes was more difficult. She did, in fact, look like a rather "sterotypical old lady." She was short and overweight, with a hairstyle and manner of dressing very typical for an older woman living on a government-subsidy income. She walked a lot, if slowly due to arthritis, and wore tennis shoes. She had a ready smile. People were inclined to patronize her in a pleasant way. She was, in fact, quite bright and well informed on a wide range of topics. She had a great sense of humor, and (revealed slowly over the first year I knew her) wrote rather charming short stories and painted attractive water colors. Her age and income status were quite limiting in the impression that she made.

With the concern about the labeling and stereotyping by others out of the way, her own negative self-evaluation came to the foreground. Mildred was seriously distressed by her chaotic and unsuccessful life. She had been bright and quite attractive as a young woman. She had worked in civil service at one time and had wanted to complete college. Instead, she had four ex-husbands and, she revealed at this point, a daughter in a neighboring state from whom she was estranged for reasons she either did not know or did not want to discuss.

She had multiple psychiatric hospital admissions and had lived on disability due to psychiatric problems most of her life. She had felt most productive and most "at home" during one admission lasting several years, when she had a responsible job in the state hospital laundry and a good relationship with one of the psychiatrists. Out of the hospital, her life had been marginal jobs (she bragged of having once been a "taxi dancer"), residential care homes or single-room-occupancy hotels, and sometimes lying about suicidal impulses or hearing voices to get back in the hospital.

Of these various concerns from her life review, the one that emerged as unresolved was her relationship with her daughter. As we explored this in more detail, it developed that she felt that family members had taken her daughter away from her. After one of her early hospitalizations, she was told by family to stay away from her daughter because she was unfit and she had obeyed them. As far as I could determine this was a family decision, without input from hospital staff and without legal sanction.

Her attempts to contact her daughter after she had come of age were generally marked by the daughter's becoming angry and Mildred's retreating. At other times, the daughter had rejected Mildred's requests for assistance of some sort (money or a place to stay). Mildred interpreted all of these interactions as personal rejection and felt quite hurt by them.

As we discussed these incidents again and again, I worked toward having Mildred try to take the point of view of her daughter: to see that the daughter had likely felt abandoned and would still feel hurt by that. She also reconstructed the kinds of things that the other family members would have told her daughter about her. Finally, we worked in some detail on what exactly she wanted from her daughter: help, forgiveness, an ideal intimate mother-daughter relationship, conversation, and various other options. After considerable work over a period of months, she decided that she wanted renewed contact, acknowledgement of relationship, a chance to visit her grandchildren, and cessation of hostilities.

We then role played her initial contacts until she felt comfortable making the phone call. To our mutual surprise, the call went rather well; after a few more calls and letters, a visit to her daughter was set up. Her anxiety rose considerably immediately before the visit, and she almost canceled. After we reviewed her skills and ways of getting in touch with me by telephone, she calmed enough to go. The visit went generally well, with only one emergency call when she was feeling rejected because the family had left her alone for an afternoon due to other plans. In a half-hour phone call, she was able to put this into perspective.

After some time consolidating these gains and increasing her social involvements elsewhere (she joined a discussion group that I ran in a senior center and also a local creative writing group), therapy tapered off. We maintained contact through the discussion group, and she would come in once every few months to discuss a problem or a crisis. The relationship went on at this level for a few years.

We had a renewed set of sessions over growing conflicts in a relationship that Mildred had developed with another woman. Mildred did housework for this woman and also socialized with her. In therapy, we would discuss both sides of the arguments they had and her responses. After a dispute over doing dishes, the relationship was broken off, and Mildred rather suddenly left town, moving several hundred miles away to live with a family in a rural county and care for their children.

Several months later, she suddenly reappeared in the discussion group with a story about discovering that the family were marijuana farmers and she had been more isolated on the farm with them than she could stand. She had also found the children much more work than anticipated. She recounted a somewhat dramatic "escape" from the farm in which she left unannounced, walked to town, and got someone in the local senior center to buy her a bus ticket back to Ventura County. With the move, she had sacrificed her subsidized housing, and her Social Security checks were missing for a couple of months because of changing her address. She handled these problems rather well, having had extensive experience with the social services system.

She returned to our clinic as well and, with more therapy visits and a mild antipsychotic, did rather well for another year. She then started having trouble with landlords, got evicted, and moved with some assistance from us. Within a few weeks, Mildred managed to get into an argument with another team member, who asked her about the wine bottles in her kitchen, and with our psychiatrist, who refused to change her schedule to see Mildred when she appeared unannounced to demand a medication refill. She then appeared in every hospital emergency room in the county and got admitted in one facility with heart trouble and to a private psychiatric facility in another county. She left that institution to live in the residential care home she liked least and specifically requested that our program not be the one to offer her follow-up care.

After a couple of years of stability, she let it be known that there was no more animosity. When I visited her to discuss using her case history, we had a pleasant chat about our contacts and she showed me a poem of hers that had been published in an anthology.

DISCUSSION

Rapport Building. When I met Mildred, she was extremely anxious. Although eager to find help, she was also quite worried about being placed in institutional care. Part of building rapport with Mildred was being willing and able to discuss her risk of being hospitalized and to examine whether such a decision was at all likely, given the problems she was having. That discussion and the favorable results of the personality test made a big impression on her and won her trust. She remarked for years afterward that I had told her she was not crazy when others thought she was and she was wondering if they were right. Once that hurdle had been leaped, we were able to begin discussing her current problems.

Techniques in Therapy. The first phase of therapy with Mildred was oriented toward very specific goals. We rehearsed assertive skills, which she had learned earlier, and discovered a way to resolve her immediate conflict with her caseworker. With that problem out of the way, the more general question of social skills and friends arose. A fairly straightforward and very specific change in her conversational style (not revealing immediately that she was a former mental patient) resulted in significant improvement in her social contacts with others. In fact, she joined a number of discussion groups and interest groups.

What she had first presented as a very similar problem with bias against older people developed into a more global issue in her own self-esteem and evaluation of her own life. In fact, the bias she experienced was her own feeling that she had aged unsuccessfully and her life had been wasted. While ageism clearly exists, and I have had clients for whom the ageist prejudice of others was a major stressor, some older adults first describe their negative feelings about the aging process or about the way their individual life stories have turned out in terms of "what life is like for older people in America." Understood as a problem with self-esteem, her concern about ageism led to a life review.

Mildred thus presents another example (along with Nora in Chapter 12) of a life review not prompted by death. In this instance, life review is clearly in response to a sense of dissatisfaction with the course of her life, with a need to reinterpret her life and alter the outcome (Butler & Lewis, 1982). More particularly, the problem-ridden relationship with her only child, and the clear sense of being unfinished with that relationship, motivated the life review in Mildred's therapy. Once she got to the point of actually visiting her daughter, she began to talk of having been motivated to tackle this lifelong problem now because of the awareness that time was running out. It is unclear to me whether this post hoc observation was accurate or was simply an attempt to answer the often unanswerable question: "Why now, why not earlier?" It is clear that Mildred had an unresolved life issue of major importance, that needed both life review and corrective action so that she could achieve some sense of completion.

One final aspect of her therapy that deserves further comment is the role that diagnosis and assessment played. In the first stage of working with Mildred, my best assessment was that she was in crisis but not psychotic. As I learned more of her life history, it became clear that she had lived a very marginally functional existence most of her adult life in spite of being bright and rather creative. To explain this fact and to understand Mildred better, I and the other team members involved with her considered various personality disorders, but found none that were entirely accurate. Toward the end of our work with her, recurrence of manic episodes would seem to substantiate a bipolar affective disorder, which we assumed had been relatively stable for the preceding 8 years. In retrospect, it would have been very helpful for Mildred had we realized this earlier in the course of working with her. However, even in retrospect we could find no reason to have suspected the diagnosis earlier than we did.

Gerontological Issues. Mildred, like the two women of the preceding chapter, illustrates the potential of working with more severely disordered older adults. Unlike Sophia and Lila, Mildred had an established history of low-level functioning and of multiple hospitalizations and long-term mental health treatment in the community. These decades of experience gave her a considerable background in various psychological techniques and psychiatric medications. She was very group-wise. While attending discussion groups, she was very helpful both by modeling good group member behavior and by the quality of her insights about other members. She was, in many ways, one of the most psychologically minded older adults with whom I have worked.

She also presented an oral history of mental health treatment. While proud of having been in civil service in her early adulthood, her highest achievement after her first hospitalization was a period of time when she had been a supervisor in one of the work units at a state psychiatric hospital—before work programs were ended by the requirement that patients be paid minimum wage. She had been one of the early group of patients returned to the community and a pioneer patient member of day-treatment programs in the local community. She knew many mental health professionals and could be quite observant and witty about those she liked, as well as those she disliked. She also had astute and mostly accurate observations about which approaches worked with her and which did not.

This lengthy period of treatment may have served to counterbalance the long duration of her disability. It seems to me that the outcome of our work together was quite positive, even though conventional wisdom would suggest that it would be futile to look for positive change in an older adult with a long history of mental disorder. However, as noted by Miller and Cohen (1987), the life course of psychotic disorders is quite varied, with many marginally functional adults showing improvement over periods of many years, and some showing improvement for the first time late in life.

While we have assumed that Mildred was manic depressive rather than schizophrenic, her level of functioning over her adult life was similar to that of persons with schizophrenic disorders, and we have little information to speak with certainty of the category of her disorder. In spite of this history, Mildred achieved significant change in her day-to-day life and also resolved a long-standing problem with her daughter as part of a life review. She even felt "freed up" to return to creative activities of painting and writing that she had learned during lengthy stays in the hospital.

One area for mutually beneficial exchange between gerontology and mental health is the understanding of the older chronically mentally ill patient. Often not recognized as a distinct group in either service system, these individuals cross between the aging services network and the mental health network and are typically misunderstood and poorly served by each system. From the gerontological viewpoint, which emphasizes a life span approach to understanding human development, one lesson is that mental health treatments may have some positive affect on such people, but it may be slowly accumulative across the many years of treatment. The relative impact of biological changes with age (Finch & Morgan, 1987), cognitive changes of aging (Niederehe & Rusin, 1987), and cohort and developmental effect (Cohler & Ferrono, 1987) all represent areas of gerontological study that may help in the understanding of the aging severely mentally ill.

Relationship Issues. Mildred had sufficient experience with mental health treatment and mental health professionals that her relationship with me was largely within this role-defined context. There were, at separate times, some hints of erotic transference and of filial transference, in which I became the idealized son she never had. The erotic elements chiefly came up as she discussed her own sexual needs and frustrations and would flirt during sessions or speculate about my abilities, as compared to those of the men she was dating. With Mildred, these feelings were kept within the bounds of reality by simply redirecting the conversation back to her needs and the problems she was experiencing with men who were available to her. I also acknowledged the basic validity of her need to be seen as a person with sexual needs.

As she focused on her relationship with her daughter, Mildred showed some signs of wishing to mother me. As one of my earliest clients, she had a certain proprietary interest in me. During this period, she would often brag, to office staff and to older adults in the community, about what I was doing and changes I was making. There was clearly an undertone that she was partly responsible for my development. She gave me advice about work and people whom she knew to be clients. In various other small ways, she showed signs of motherly affection.

When she actually planned and made the visit to her daughter, there was a certain sense of her placing me in the role of the son with whom she was close, who was helping her with the daughter from whom she was estranged. In general, I think that these transferential elements were helpful to the progress she made. The actual behaviors were at times mildly disconcerting, since being mothered by a client is incongruous for an (at that time) early-30s male professional in the first years of post-Ph.D. experience who did not take mothering particularly well from his own mother. Understanding what was happening in transferential terms as part of the therapy probably kept me from inappropriately rejecting some of these behaviors as she was practicing her mothering skills prior to using them with her daughter.

Regarding countertransference: After the first couple of months of therapy, my feelings about Mildred were always positive, even as I wondered what her level of disability and her diagnosis were. This positive feeling for her was helpful in motivating me to work with a potentially difficult client and keeping me involved with her through some difficult times. In retrospect, I think it hampered me in two ways. Even though she had shared some early history of drug abuse, I never really pursued the theme of substance abuse with her and specifically did not seriously consider whether she was drinking heavily in the present. The other way in which this positive feeling may have hampered me is that I might have been more active in confronting her about the signs of developing mania earlier than I did. It is impossible to say whether either of these changes would have made a difference; but my experience with Mildred has taught me a valuable lesson about the importance of ongoing assessment with clients for whom you have strong positive feelings and the motivation to normalize their apparent problems.

Summary. Mildred provides a valuable lesson in the potential for change in an individual with a long-term history of mental disorder and a lifelong pattern of marginal functioning. For several years she benefited from therapy and resolved some major issues in her life. She also had a significant relapse after this period of therapy. While the relapse was clearly a major setback, it did not completely erase the gains she had established earlier. In fact, it may well have served to rebalance her life at lower, and therefore more comfortable and stable, levels of achievement and intimacy (cf. Lamb, 1987).

Conclusion:
A Maturity-Based Model for Psychotherapy With Older Adults

The writing of this book has been an educational experience for me in that the case history method has made some old ideas much more vivid and has led to some new discoveries about the nature of psychotherapy with older adults. In this concluding chapter, these discoveries are described in ascending order of abstraction. That is, the first several observations will be about specific themes in psychotherapy with older adults: the interconnectedness of their problems, counseling about chronic illness and disability, counseling about grief and dying, prescribing activity and social involvement for the older client, and the role of life review in psychotherapy with older adults. These topical issues will be followed by observations on psychotherapeutic intimacy with older clients and on ethical issues in work with older adults.

The concluding section presents some initial thoughts on what a psychotherapy that is grounded in late life, rather than in childhood, might look like. My early education in psychotherapy with older adults involved readings that were grounded in a loss-deficit model of aging. Early authors explicitly argued that aging involved deterioration of functioning and regression to second childhood, and was characterized by losses (Berezin, 1963; Gitelson, 1948). These early views are generally rationalized in terms of unavoidable biological decline, and in the traditional psychodynamic view of old age as regression to increased dependency. Even in more recent writing in family systems theory (e.g., Walsh, 1988), there is the assumption that late life is primarily a time of losses. The concept of loss is very general, in my view overgeneralized, and includes death of friends, loss of physical ability, retirement, children growing up and leaving home, reduced income, and so on.

The increased knowledge about gerontology, and the increasing interest in psychotherapy with the elderly in the past couple of decades, can be viewed as encouraging the application of therapeutic approaches developed with younger adults to the elderly, and as encouraging a skepticism about the universality of losses and deficit in late life. The first part of this chapter reflects the themes of optimism about the outcomes of therapy with older adults and providing specific interventions for specific problems of late life. In the second part, the lessons from gerontology described in the Introduction are combined with the lessons from these case histories to outline a maturity model of late life.

Interconnectedness of Problems. My original intent in writing this book was to describe cases that would illustrate the themes and content areas described in *Psychotherapy with Older Adults*. It proved impossible to find cases that exemplify one and only one topic or content area in doing therapy with older adults. Cases that at first seemed to me to be about depression have proved to involve caregivers and grieving. Cases selected to exemplify grieving have involved the client's adjustment to disability as well as to the loss of loved ones. Cases about relationships have involved death and grief. A case about sexuality involved a man who was successfully being treated for manic-depressive disorder. The list could go on and on, but the point is that topical presentations about the problems of older adults including my own (Knight, 1986, 1989) either miss or misrepresent a primary reality of late life: Older adults have multiple problems, and pure cases are hard, if not impossible, to find. Working with older adults in psychotherapy tends to involve multiple problems, all of which are challenging. In most cases, these multiple problems will include issues generally seen as outside of the domain of psychotherapy: health problems and social service problems.

CONTENT ISSUES IN
PSYCHOTHERAPY WITH THE ELDERLY

Health Psychology and Rehabilitation Counseling. Continued work with older adults and the writing of these case histories have made more and more clear to me that much of working with emotionally distressed older adults involves working with older adults who are chronically ill and/or physically disabled and struggling to adjust to these problems. If the ages and the life stories were deleted, this volume could be understood as a collection of stories about people struggling with blindness, impaired ambulation, cancer, chronic heart disease, emphysema, diabetes, and chronic mental disorders. In setting out to do psychological work with older adults in a community-based mental health setting, I have found myself learning about these illnesses and their psychological impact, learning about pain control, learning about adherence to medical treatment, learning about rehabilitation strategies, and learning to assess behavioral signs of medication reactions. This work has taken me into hospitals, nursing homes, cardiac rehabilitation programs, emergency rooms, and to the bedside of many severely disabled older adults.

In doing this work, I have become acquainted with physicians and nurses and have learned how to talk to them and with them. I have learned much about the limitations of medicine and about the demands that patients place on doctors. I have learned to think about hospitals and other medical settings as organizational systems inhabited by human beings, but operating within distinctive social rules. I have come to better appreciate my own expertise by observing that many people with medical training are as uncomfortable with emotionality, psychosis, and suicidal threats as I am with blood, physical symptoms, and medical emergencies.

This aspect of working with older adults involves specialized knowledge and specialized skills, compared to other areas of psychotherapeutic practice where physical problems and the physical dimension of the person can be more safely ignored. The increased proportion of chronic illness and disability with each decade of life, and the increased correlation of the physical and the psychological in later life, make it impossible to function without the ability to discuss physical problems and understand when a problem may have physical causes. This principle does not mean that every psychotherapist working with the elderly must be a physician. It does mean that we must be able to talk intelligently and cooperatively with physicians and with older clients who need to discuss the very real physical problems that they face.

The goals of such therapy are most often oriented to an accurate understanding of the client's functional ability, an acceptance of real deficits in function, and a search for ways to optimize functioning given those real disabilities. The first of these goals is often very elusive. The best available medical diagnoses and rehabilitation assessments may leave the psychotherapist and the client none too clear about what the true level of functioning is. Often the client's assessment of his or her abilities will be ongoing trial and error. This process must be guided by the best available information *and* by the potential costs of being wrong: relapse and rehospitalization, pain, excess dependency, depression, and so on.

Adjustment to lost ability requires confronting the disability and grieving for it. This work is not as optimistic as encouraging younger adults who are not disabled to try new activities or new strategies in relationships. Many therapists new to work with the aged find themselves nearly unable to speak such sentences as, "Mrs. G., you are not going to get your vision back. You must have some feelings about that." On the other hand, therapeutic experience with the disabled makes it easier to say the words, and makes the work more hopeful once you have seen that this is the beginning of improvement in mood, if not in vision.

Much writing and discussion about the elderly is based on a loss-deficit model and argues that the work of therapy with the elderly is adjusting to the natural losses of late life and grieving for them. This model is wrong on two counts: First, there is nothing especially *natural* about blindness or heart disease or cancer. The fact that they happen more frequently to older adults does not make these diseases and disabilities part of normal development. It certainly does not make the individual older person experience these problems either as normal or as less of a crisis than they would be for a younger adult.

Second, the loss-deficit model fails to suggest the next step of optimizing functioning. Rehabilitation may start by accepting the deficit in functioning but it does not end there. The next step is to consider how life may be improved. The goal may not necessarily be a return to premorbid levels of functioning and mood; but there is always room for improvement over the initial level of mood and functioning. Applying a modification of the Lewinsohn & MacPhillamy (1974) and Lewinshon et al. (1978) pleasant events model, the therapist can maximize the enjoyment of life by increasing activities that the patient has enjoyed and which he or she is still able to do. This work may also include approximating some old activities or finding new ways to accomplish the same ends. While the goal description is easy, this work is often highly emotional and full of resistance in the traditional therapeutic sense. What the client typically wants is to not have the disability. This fact will be confronted over and over in the process of improving the quality of life.

Working with disabled clients also raises the home visit question in a very practical way. Perhaps the most compelling reason to do psychotherapy in the home is that disabled people cannot come to the office for therapy, or can get there only at considerable cost of effort, time, and pain. To insist that therapy be available only in the office is to exclude many individuals who need the comfort and the change available in therapy. Unfortunately, there are many therapists who will not leave their offices to see clients (about which more will be said in a later section), and many third-party payers (including Medicare and Medicaid) regularly refuse to pay for home visit psychotherapy.

The role of mind and body in uniting to make up daily human experience is perhaps nowhere more regularly evident than in working with older adults. Consider the stories in this volume: Frances ignored her diabetes and construed some of its effects as anxiety; Lana and Nora changed emotional feelings into physical symptoms, but also got sick from time to time and ignored those real signs of physical frailty; neither Agnes nor her physician was certain whether her shortness of breath was anxiety or a symptom of medical illness. The ambiguity of such instances can be unsettling; but the intellectual challenge and the opportunity to learn daily how the mind affects the body, and the body in turn affects the mind, are stimulating and enlightening.

Death, Dying, and Grief. Talking about death and grief seem to me to be central to therapy whenever the need arises. In training new therapists to work with older adults, I have been struck by the great difficulty many of them have with this topic. Some therapists fail to hear it come up in therapy sessions, fail to perceive it as a major issue, or take the client's reluctance to discuss the issue as a sign that grieving has been resolved. When I have presented these cases in classes, the emotional reaction of listeners has served as a clue to me that familiarity with this topic has blinded me to how difficult it is for others to stay with discussing grief and the loss of loved ones.

There is, of course, a general social prohibition against talking about death and dying in our society. Added to this, for most younger adults, any confrontation with death or conversation about death is "off time" in the Neugarten and Hagestad (1976) sense. That is, if younger therapists were not working with older adults (or other people who are facing death), they might not confront the reality of death and dying and the loss of persons close to them for a decade or more. Being "on time" does not necessarily make it easier. Middle-aged adults, who are themselves facing the issue for the first time, may have difficulty precisely because it is a current and unresolved issue in their own psychological lives. Experiential preparation for such work is an essential part of learning to work with older adults and is important for all psychotherapists. After all, not all people die "on time" either.

The training to do such work is technically simple. Therapists need some knowledge of the typical psychological and social course of preparing to die and of grief for others. Mostly they need to learn the skill of listening comfortably, and of keeping clients talking about an issue that both client and therapist find uncomfortable. In Larry McMurtry's *Lonesome Dove* (1985), one of the cowboys dies crossing a river. The Captain expresses the usual human conviction that the rest of the crew needs to get their minds off the death. Augustus replies: "Wrong theory. Talk will kill it. Anything gets boring if you talk about it long enough, even death."

Death plays a different role in working with the elderly than I expected when I started this work more than a decade ago. I thought working with older adults would involve much counseling in the preparing-to-die mode. For the most part, I have found people over the age of 70 to be already at peace with their own eventual death. I have come to understand the struggle with accepting one's own death to be a task for the middle-aged, and perhaps the young-old, rather than a developmental task of late life. On the other hand, grief work is very common: Grieving for spouses, siblings, parents, friends, children, and pets is a major part of psychological work with older adults. This grief work often involves multiple deaths in a short period of time and can also involve working through unresolved griefs from years, even decades ago.

I have also discovered in a very immediate way the essential unpredictability of death. I have seen many older clients who appeared close to death when I first met them. They were physically extremely frail, often with life-threatening conditions, and quite frequently dependent on tubes, catheters, oxygen tanks, and so on. Many of them are still alive today, and still physically very frail and looking very near death. Most of these people are less depressed or less anxious than when our work started and are therefore noticeably more functional.

The healthy active clients have often been the ones who died. People not known to be ill have died. Clients who saw a doctor occasionally and took medication, but were not disabled or functionally impaired, have simply died between one appointment and the next. I have worked with physically frail older adults (for example, Rose, in this volume) whose children have suddenly and unexpectedly died.

I have also known clients who wanted very much to die, whose bodies simply go on working. In contrast, I have known those who want very much to live who have died. The unpredictability and uncontrollability of death have been difficult lessons to learn. I have at times been saddened, angry, and simply baffled by the capriciousness of death as it impacts our lives. I have generally had the great fortune to have worked with colleagues who talked about death and dying, who would listen to me talk about it, and who would make me talk about it when I didn't want to or when I blandly assured them that I was "just fine."

The somewhat peculiar stance that many therapists and other helping professionals have toward suicide in the elderly is quite likely rooted in our own difficulty in thinking about death and in confronting the other problems of later life. In the abstract, suicide can seem like a way of controlling death. We can make death predictable and expectable by taking our own life. In the concrete instance, especially with people who decide to talk to a therapist about suicide, most people turn to suicide in depression and despair, hoping to be talked out of it.

Since the problems of the elderly often seem depressing and overwhelming to the young and the middle aged, many younger adults will too readily see suicide as a comprehensible option for the elderly. In my clinical experience, the elderly often have more strength to deal with the problems of late life than do the young, and often discover solutions and find rewards in life that I did not anticipate. It is one thing to think in the abstract that "I would rather kill myself than face going blind"; once you discover and accept progressive blindness, there can be many reasons to go on living. This is one of many clinical experiences that have led me to suspect that the elderly are in meaningful ways more mature than those of us who are younger, a topic I will return to later in this chapter.

Life Review. In a related vein, I have discovered while writing up these cases, a strong relationship between the use of life review and the process of therapeutic grief work that I had not suspected. Almost every instance in this book where life review is a major part of the therapy is a case that involves grieving for the loss of a loved one. The life review was itself largely motivated by unresolved grief from previous losses and by the need to review what life had been with the deceased in order to comprehend what life could be like without the deceased. Even preparation for one's own death often has had a more future-oriented theme: The dying person may examine unfinished business and question what needs to be done before dying; the survivor reviews life in order to find some sense in the loss of the loved one and, more difficult, reason for a life without the loved one.

The major exception in this volume is Lana. In her case, life review seemed motivated by a realization of the role of emotion in her life and the need to understand why the expression of feeling had been frustrated and suppressed, as well as what life would be like had she been more in touch with her emotions. In this instance, life review is engaged in as a means to the integration of a new point of view about life.

The same might be said of Mildred, who engaged in life review in a struggle to find an improved self-concept and identify major unfinished issues in her life. Her example is perhaps the most typically Eriksonian use of life review; however, Mildred is probably not the sort of client Erikson had in mind.

The collection of examples in this volume suggests to me a more narrowly defined role for life review in working with older adults. Rather than being a general prescription for adjustment to the later years, it is perhaps better understood as part of the grieving process and, in some instances, as a part of integrating new knowledge gained in therapy into the client's self-schema. The first use is, I suspect, problem-specific rather than age-specific. The role of life review in integrating new concepts into one's theory of the self is likely to occur at any age when a radically new perspective is gained on one's own life.

This suggests that life review may have a fairly limited role in psychotherapy with older adults, but a very prominent role in grief counseling. This statement does not apply to reminiscence as a general phenomenon nor does it apply to the psychoeducational use of autobiographical techniques (e.g., Birren & Deutchman, 1990), which are often quite beneficial and enjoyable, but are not essentially psychotherapeutic in the treatment sense.

Activity, Activities, and Older Adults. I have been struck by how much of the therapeutic effort described in this book has been focused on encouraging people to be less active. In working with Elaine and Warren, Rose, Jerry and Bea, and Nora, a major part of therapy was encouraging the client to moderate activity, to choose more enjoyable activity, or to focus on friendship or family rather than activity. It seems that much of rehabilitation counseling has been encouraging people to monitor their activities and to carefully select a few activities that they will enjoy. Often a major part of counseling has been to encourage clients to feel good about doing less. In many instances, another motivation for reducing activity has been to increase time available to spend with spouse and other family. As noted in the Introduction, this is consistent with recent trends in understanding life satisfaction in later life.

In general, however, it seems that family and professionals often naively advocate for high levels of activity and involvement in formal group activities. As seen in this volume, increased happiness may often lie in surrendering unpleasant activities and freeing up time to spend with loved ones. When the goal is the improvement of the client's general mood level, suggested changes need to focus on what is pleasurable for that individual person and, more generally, on what activities or social contacts involve contact with confidants with whom one has a pleasant relationship. As seen in the Introduction, formal activities, contact with acquaintances, and contacts with critical and argumentative family members often lead to increased depression.

Even when part of the solution for an older person's problems involves casework or increased socialization, it should not be too readily assumed that the problem has no psychological component. Practical solutions to the problems of the elderly are, in general, sufficiently obvious that the older person, their family, or other service providers will have thought of such answers well before the client sees a psychotherapist. These previous attempts to solve the problem should be explored, and the reasons for their failures may be very instructive in setting goals for the therapy.

Many of the cases discussed in this volume (e.g., Helen, Rose, Frances, Mildred) resulted in increased contact with senior recreation centers and/or volunteer projects in the community. These social connections occurred only after several weeks of psychotherapy, which worked through the client's individualized resistance to social contact, often based on failed experiences trying to pursue activities that had never been enjoyable.

This type of work requires some knowledge of the social world of the elderly, which does not have to be extraordinarily extensive but does need to go beyond the commonly believed, but entirely false assumptions of many younger adults. The assumption that living in an age-segregated environment will lead to increased friendships is something that only a naive outsider to that world can believe. Many age-segregated environments are very intolerant of frailty and of social deviance of any sort (cf. Frankfather, 1977).

Each senior recreation center and meal site tends to have its own particular social ecology. Recommending that clients go to such places to find activity or friendship is risky if you do not know the particular range of activity or the degree of openness to newcomers at that site. In one locale in which I have worked, the range of settings went from one site, which attracted retired professionals with a wide range of activities, to another, which mostly served former state hospital patients and had an environment similar to the day room in a chronic ward. Often part of initial rapport building has been showing that I understand and agree with the client's perception of why finding appropriate activity or help has been so difficult.

While this understanding is not terribly difficult to acquire, the lack of it among psychotherapists working with a general population may be one reason why older adults can seem difficult to understand. The formal network of health and social services for older adults, and the formal distinctions between different levels, can be learned in a lecture or two. Some informal visiting at such places can do a great deal toward providing a more experiential framework for understanding the environments of the elderly. These environments are unfamiliar territory for most younger adults.

We acquire some experience of school, work, military, sports, and family settings through our own lives, and this forms a background for understanding what other clients tell us. The settings of the elderly (senior recreation centers, retirement hotels, hospitals, nursing homes, doctors' offices, senior meal sites, volunteer programs, mobile home parks) are unfamiliar ground for most adults, including psychotherapists. Unfortunately, we often seem to confuse this unfamiliarity with the settings of older adults with inability to understand the older adults themselves. When older adults tell us strange things about the settings in which they live, we should perhaps be more ready to trust our psychotherapeutic skills in understanding others and in working within the client's point of view.

Home Visits and Psychotherapy with the Elderly. My own thinking on the use of home visits in psychotherapy with the elderly is the fairly radical position that whether therapy occurs in the office or in the home is largely irrelevant (cf. Knight, 1986, 1989). The decision, it seems to me, depends quite simply on whether it is easier for the therapist to go to the client or for the client to come to the therapist. To illustrate this point, I have written these case histories without reference (in most of them) to whether visits occurred in the office, the client's home, or both. Major parts of therapy with John, Sophia, Elaine and Warren, and Frances occurred in their homes. Some sessions with Rose, Rena, and Helen were in their homes. In my experience, there has been no great increase in dependency, no loss of role definition, and no noticeable decline in the effectiveness of psychotherapy when sessions move to the client's home.

There is some need to be more active in defining one's role when doing home visits. It is perhaps easier for the client to think that you are like a nurse, pastor, caseworker, or salesman. On the whole, it seems to me that these confusions are more obvious and more accessible when doing home visits, but also occur in the office without the therapist's knowing about them. Interruptions are more common in the home setting and must be coped with. Privacy issues can become very important and may require some planning to assure that visits can take place when privacy is possible. These changes seem minimal and unimportant next to the consideration of denying therapy either to the homebound or to those who are so physically frail that travel to the office is an extreme hardship. This denial of mental health services is, at this writing, codified in Medicare and Medicaid regulations that are based on the assumption that psychotherapy is only effective in certain physical settings.

This belief that psychotherapy works in the office but not elsewhere is often identified with the professional discipline of the therapist. On the whole, psychologists and psychiatrists are unwilling to make home visits, and social workers and nurses are willing to do so. In fact, much of my career as a manager of multidisciplinary teams has been spent encouraging psychologists and psychiatrists to do more home visits, and encouraging nurses and social workers to have more clients come to the office. In training new therapists, one often encounters almost magical beliefs that they have more power, status, or role security when they are in the clinic rather than the home. In my thinking it is just as curious to assume that one has therapeutic power when one is in an office setting as it is to assume that those powers decrease when one steps outside.

THERAPEUTIC
INTIMACY WITH OLDER CLIENTS:
EFFECT ON THE THERAPIST

Counseling with older adults seems to confront the therapist with a different set of clinical problems and with clients who elicit different needs and personal issues from the therapist. The emotional reactions seem to be stronger in work with older adults than in individual work with other clients. It seems to me to be comparable to the need to be clear about one's own family dynamics in order to work in conjoint family therapy (Hall, 1981; Simon, 1988). Unfortunately, whereas family therapists have been quick to realize this tendency and are prolific in writing about it, there is relatively little commentary on this problem in the literature on psychotherapy and aging.

I have included in each chapter some of my own personal response to each person. Genevay and Katz's *Countertransference and Older Clients* (1990) provides a variety of personal reactions from others with clinical and social service experience with the elderly. This can serve as a guideline for others who will, of course, have other personal issues and differing familial experience with the elderly to deal with. In addition to this very personal need to separate unfinished business with older family members, and one's own fears of aging and death, from working with older adults in therapy, there are some general reactions to working with the elderly that deserve summary and comment.

The problems faced by older adults are often seen as more real and more overwhelming than those of younger clients. This recognition is often experienced by the younger therapist as a sense of heaviness or even despair. Older clients confront us with the reality of chronic illness and the real possibility of the death of those we love, and the therapist often finds this depressing and overwhelming. It can be difficult to separate one's own emotional reaction to these problems from those of the client.

It can also be difficult for therapists new to working with the elderly to confront such issues directly. Being unwilling to talk about a client's grief, disability, progressive loss of vision, and so forth is generally the therapist's problem. The therapist may feel that such problems are best ignored. The client does not actually have the option of ignoring the problem and needs someone to talk to. As discussed in several chapters in this book, such interventions leave the client equally disabled as before the therapy, but often less depressed.

Addressing these issues will benefit the clients and will change the therapist as well. Working with older adults has compelled me to resolve personal emotional issues about my parents that I otherwise would have ignored for another decade or two. It has given me a sense of the reality and unexpectedness of death and chronic illness that I do not find in friends close to my age. Being able to assist clients with multiple devastating problems has given me a confidence in the power of psychotherapy that I have not seen in other practitioners. There are rewards in doing therapy with older adults, but there are painful realities to confront as well.

ETHICAL ISSUES IN PSYCHOTHERAPY WITH OLDER ADULTS

A common topic in therapy with older adults will be the client's deciding to die or deciding to discontinue treatment that would prolong life. Such decisions are, of course, intensely personal and value laden. My personal ethic has been to encourage exploration of the question without encouraging any particular solution. As was seen with Agnes and with Bea, this position often ended with the client deciding in favor of a natural death and then changing her mind and seeking treatment. These cases clearly speak to the extreme ambivalence that the client experiences when faced with such a decision. It is my perception that these decisions could easily have been influenced by the therapist's values. It troubles me that many people have clear-cut positions on such issues, feeling either that a natural death is always better or that everyone should be encouraged to live.

I have also seen such decisions strongly affected by family members who convey, implicitly or explicitly, that their lives would be either easier or more difficult if the ill person were to die. Family members generally have conflicting interests in such situations and often have differing values. I am certain in my own mind that I have seen families express sufficient distress about the possibility of prolonged dependency and caregiving that an already depressed patient has chosen to die rather than be a burden to the family. I have also seen people who were very tired of living struggle to hang on because other family members were very dependent on them emotionally. The discussion of such issues could benefit from a psychological and family systems perspective. Therapists also need to be trained to keep their personal values out of an already complex and volatile situation.

The family systems perspective also raises an interesting ethical issue in therapy with the elderly. When caregiving is an issue, whose needs should predominate? An individual approach leads to the therapist's advocating for the individual needs of whichever family member has come to the office. A family systems approach would encourage getting more people into the office and working toward a compromise solution. I often use an exercise in class in which a family conference is role played by the students and then the question is posed: How would your intervention have been different if you had seen only one of these people? How would the intervention have differed if you had seen only certain subsets of this family group? The underlying values question (Who should be seen before the assessment is finished?) is largely unanswerable, but it seems essential that everyone working with older adults worry about the question continually.

Confidentiality and control of therapy issues with older adults receive too little attention in work with the elderly. In all sorts of settings, older adults are assumed to have less right to confidentiality than younger adults. Family members especially are often included in discussions and may be consulted routinely about what step to take next. Unless the older person is cognitively incompetent, such behavior is inexcusable. Older adults have as much right to privacy and to determine their own goals in therapy as anyone else. It has also been my experience that there is no problem in most instances in getting the appropriate consent.

There are, of course, times when people understand what you want to do and disagree. That seems to happen with younger adults as well!

SUMMARY:
TOWARD A MATURITY-BASED
PSYCHOTHERAPY

I have been studying and writing about psychotherapy with older adults for about 15 years. For most of that time, I have argued that therapy with the elderly is different, both in terms of content areas covered and in the nature of the therapeutic relationship. I have also generally argued that the goals, techniques, and process of therapy are not necessarily different with older adults.

There are some areas of needed specialized knowledge and experience. Assessment issues are more complex with the elderly; and some ability to distinguish among health problems, psychological problems, and social service needs is essential. Some ability to distinguish between dementing illnesses and normal aging is imperative. An understanding of the social world of the elderly is of great importance. Finally, and perhaps most difficult, the therapist needs to be comfortable working with the elderly. This comfort requires being at peace with one's own family issues about aging, confronting countertransference about older family members, and being comfortable with talking about chronic illness, disability, and death with people who are experiencing these major life problems.

Why Aren't Older People More Depressed? Gerontology as a discipline has often been split between researchers, who have kept discovering that aging is a more positive experience than society is presumed to believe it is, and practitioners, who have struggled with the problems of some of the elderly and have painted a dismal picture of aging. The loss-deficit model of aging, which portrays the normative course of later life as a series of losses and the typical response as depression, is an integral part of the practitioner heritage.

A series of recent discoveries tends to undermine that picture. Retirement and the empty-nest marriage have been found to be related to increases in life satisfaction for most older adults. Life satisfaction seems to be stable over the adult life span (Costa et al., 1987). The NIMH Catchment Area Studies find lower prevalence rates of depression and other mental disorder in older adults as compared to younger adults (Myers et al., 1984). Gatz and Hurwicz (1990), in a cross-sectional study with a large sample, failed to find higher rates of depression among older adults; in fact, scores on depressed mood were higher for the youngest group. They did find some decrease in life satisfaction for the oldest group (past age 70).

As a clinician, the question I most often find myself asking about clients is, "Why aren't they more depressed?" To me as a younger adult, the problems seem more real and more overwhelming than those that I and most of my age-mates face and get upset about. Years of nearly exclusive work with older adults often leaves me wondering what it is that younger adults are so upset about. Every client's problem must be evaluated within the context of his or her developmental level and the tasks facing him or her. However, after spending years discussing the death of loved ones and the confronting of chronic, progressive disease, it becomes difficult to be empathic with a younger adult who is distraught because his or her parents disapprove of his or her choice of job or mate.

With the accumulation of clinical experience, my conclusion has grown stronger over the years that older adults are, in fact, more mature than younger adults (myself included) in some significant ways. Most immediately apparent in the psychotherapeutic relationship is the greater acceptance of the finitude of life and a greater comfort in talking about death. There is also the wealth of observations of people and relationships, which forms the basis of a fairly well-developed implicit personality theory for many older people. To go further with the notion requires a return to theoretical and research gerontology.

Evidence of Increasing Maturity Through Adulthood. In the *Psychotherapy* book (Knight, 1986), I discussed Neugarten's (1977) contention that there is an increase in interiority with age, where interiority is a tendency to turn inward, to become more reflective, psychologically oriented, and philosophical about life. In that earlier book, I observed that this tendency would make older adults more ready for psychotherapy. In the Introduction of this volume, several lines of evidence for more complex cognitive and emotional functioning in later years was discussed.

Although speed of processing and other components of fluid intelligence decrease with age, crystal intelligence likely remains stable. On the qualitative front, there have been suggestions of the development of expert systems, dependent on the individual's experiences in adult life (Rybash et al., 1986) and of movement to a stage of post-formal reasoning, with an appreciation of the dialectical nature of argument and perhaps of social change, and a greater appreciation of the possibility of people holding differing points of view (Rybash et al., 1986).

On the emotional side, older adults have been seen as becoming less impulsive and driven by anxiety (Gynther, 1979), more emotionally complex, with more complex reactions to events (Schulz, 1982) and more complex experience of and ability to control emotional states (Labouvie-Vief, DeVoe, & Bulka, 1989). De Rivera (1984) argued for the development of a greater range of emotions and greater experience of the transformation of emotions as a likely outcome of increased experience throughout life.

Increased androgyny (Bengtson et al., 1985; Gutmann, 1987) can also be seen as increased psychological maturity. As one moves into the second half of life, behavior and social skills can become less constricted by sex role stereotypes and therefore more fully human. At least in the context of heterosexual relationships, men and women learn skills and behaviors from one another over a period of decades.

The mechanism for such improvement can be as simple (and as complex) as the accumulation of life experiences, which can be understood as an increasingly complex database of human interaction. Breytspraak (1984) summarizes sociological and social psychological thought on the development of the self and notes that social comparison processes, reflected appraisals, and the role of person-environment interactions provide input for a dynamically evolving self-concept. Assuming that such input is continual throughout life implies that with increasing years, there is at least the potential for greater self-knowledge and the development of a more complex self.

Attacking the same notion from a somewhat different theoretical position, Bowen's family systems theory (cf. Hall, 1981) relates the development of the differentiated self to experience with one's family context. Bowen's concept of multigenerational transmission implies a general consistency from family of origin to family of marriage. Working with older families drives home the point that all older adults have experience of several family constellations: the family of origin, the family of marriage and small children, the extending family with adult children and grandchildren, and the dispersed family of later life. If one adds the knowledge gained of the spouse's family and the families of the spouses of the client's children, every older person can be something of an expert on family dynamics.

In summary, these trends in gerontological thinking suggest a potential for continual growth toward maturity throughout the adult life span. In this sense, maturity means increasing cognitive complexity, possibly including postformal reasoning; development of expertise in areas of experiential competence including work, family, and relationships; androgyny, at least in the sense of acquiring role competencies and interests stereotypically associated with the opposite gender; and a greater emotional complexity and better comprehension and control of emotional reactions.

None of the above should be taken as denying the very real problems of late life and the serious losses that some individuals face in old age. The life stories in this volume should be adequate evidence that I have no desire to gloss over the very serious challenges that face the elderly. On the other hand, this sketch of a developing model of maturity suggests the source of the strengths that older adults bring to coping with the challenges of late life.

Baltes and Baltes (1990) have proposed a selective optimization with compensation model for successful aging. In their view, older adults have both developmental and illness-imposed limitations, which require that specific areas of desired competency be selected. Older adults are often not functioning at full capability, and so the selected areas of competency can be optimized by practice, exercise, and so on. Furthermore, lost or lessened abilities can often be replaced by compensating strengths. In a similar

Elements of Maturity	Specific Challenges
Cognitive complexity	Chronic illnesses
Postformal reasoning	Disabilities
Emotional complexity	Preparation for dying
Androgeny	Grieving for loved ones
Expertise	
Areas of competency	
Multiple family experiences	
Accumulated interpersonal skills	

Figure 1. The Maturity-Specific Challenge Model

vein, the argument advanced here for psychotherapy is that the loss-deficit model be replaced by a maturity-specific challenge model. In this view, older adults are seen as mature and strong individuals who are facing specific challenges, which occur more frequently in late life and are daunting for everyone in our culture. Figure 1 summarizes the Maturity-Specific Challenge Model.

Cautions and Limitations. This view of adult development and aging as maturation in the fullest sense is not entirely new. For differing reasons, Jung (1933) and Maslow (1970) saw the second half of life as full of potential for maturation. In one of his most neglected passages, Maslow noted that most of his "self-actualized" people were older and he argued that college students did not have sufficient life experience to be self-actualized (Maslow, 1970).

A serious limitation to the benefits of maturation is posed by the effects of cohort membership and social change. Much of social gerontology could be summarized as the discovery that we consistently attribute to the aging process differences between the old and the young that are due to cohort effects. Cohort differences are due to membership in a birth-year-defined group that is socialized to certain beliefs, attitudes, and personality dimensions that will stay constant for us as we age and distinguish us from those born earlier and later.

For example, later-born cohorts in twentieth-century America have more years of formal schooling than earlier-born groups. As another example, people who matured during World War II, those who matured during the Vietnam War, and those who matured without a major military involvement will tend to have differing attitudes toward government, politics, and military actions. People will also tend to be relatively more at ease with technology in place as they mature than with technology developed in the later part of their lives. Social change occurring before or during our childhood years may be taken for granted; that occurring during our adult years will be truly experienced as change.

These cohort differences are the reasons that older people seem "old fashioned." Cohort effects and social change can also explain many of the misunderstandings that occur between young and old adults, even some of the differences in understanding between old and young within a family. While many differences within families are due to family conflicts that are normative and unavoidable, other disagreements may arise because families are composed of members of various cohorts. Becoming acquainted with members of other birth-year cohorts who are not relatives can be very helpful in separating out cohort differences from other types of family disputes.

These differences, while not developmental, are real. Working with older adults involves learning something of the folkways of members of earlier-born cohorts, just as working with adolescents or young adults demands staying current in their folkways and worldview. During times of rapid social and technological change (the twentieth century comes to mind), cohort effects may overwhelm advantages of developmental maturation for some purposes. Earlier-born adults are offended by and afraid of levels of crime and threat in the cities that persons born in my cohort and later take for granted. Changes in the role of women and in the family structure may be envied or despised but not taken for granted. Understanding *aging* is about understanding maturation, working with *old people* is about understanding people who matured in a different era.

Another important caution in understanding the maturity model is that people can, of course, grow older without growing more mature. Some people have 70 years of experience; others have one year of experience 70 times! Just as there are children in young adult bodies and adolescents in middle-aged bodies, there will be children, adolescents, and middle-aged people in old bodies. This psychological fact is, in part, the business of psychotherapy. To help such people, psychotherapists will have to learn to think past young adulthood and middle age as the goals of development.

Toward a Prospective Model for Psychotherapy. Existing models of personality begin with child development and extend to early adulthood, with some generalizations to middle age and even young old age. The principles of psychotherapy approaches based on personality models are all rooted in the concept that problems go back to faulty childhood development or to problems in the family of origin. Behavioral and cognitive therapies are obvious exceptions, but also generally confine their analyses to problems, rather than analyzing the person.

Since most patients in therapy have been relatively young adults, they are quite likely to be struggling with issues that began in childhood and in the family of origin. In fact, they have not had enough additional life experience to have problems that *could* have begun later. Theories of the person and of personal change based on young adult clients have of necessity been *retrospective* theories, relating adult life experience to experiences of childhood. In fact, freeing oneself from perceptions of life that are rooted in childhood, and from the emotional politics of one's family of origin, are principal developmental tasks of adolescence and early adulthood.

Psychotherapeutic work with older adults suggests that problems can start later in life. People may have unresolved conflicts with accepting death. The death of a spouse not properly grieved for when the client was middle-aged may complicate grief for a child in late life (Rena). Unresolved conflicts with children of a mid-life marriage may complicate caregiving arrangements in later life (Elaine and Warren). Unresolved issues with adult children and their spouses may make later years more lonely (Nora, Lana). While some problems of later life may have roots in childhood (e.g., Frances, Rose) others may have roots in the early adult years (Rena), middle age (Fred, Elaine), or even during the young-old years (JoAnn, Harold). Given a life-span view of maturation, development may become conflictual or arrested at any point in the adult life span. Given the recognition that each person is a member of several family systems during a full life span,

relationship problems can originate in the family of procreation
or in the extended family of adult children and in-laws as well as
in the family of origin.

The possibility of increasing maturity in normal development
also suggests the possibility of a *prospective* view of the life span.
The prospective view would work from a description of normative or optimal old age and try to guide adult life toward the future achievement of full maturity. While such a model cannot yet
be described fully, the possibility is clearly developing. That
model would quit trying to fit the elderly into theories and therapies developed on the young, and instead would assist the young
in learning how to be fully mature in late life.

The application of the prospective view of the life span to work
with younger adults would move beyond assuming that psychological health is defined as freedom from the problems of one's
family of origin and from childhood conflicts and perceptions.
Such work is essential to the psychological health of those who
have unfinished business in earlier stages of development, but, in
this life-span view of maturity, would not be defined as freedom
from the past but rather as preparation for the future.

Younger adults (including the middle-aged and perhaps the
young-old) could be encouraged to think about the length of the
adult life span, the role of both work and the postretirement life-
style within the total span of their lives, and the interrelationship
of the various family systems in which they will live. In this view,
current adjustment to work and home would be viewed not only
in relationship to one's past accomplishments and past family
roles but also in terms of preparation for the future.

The elements of such preparation are contained in questions
rather than answers:

- Is the current set of work and leisure activities well-balanced
  enough to support a satisfying retirement life?
- Should current disagreements with children and their spouses be
  resolved as part of planning for a mutually supportive late life family system?
- Are there relationships that need further work before one of us dies?
- Am I prepared to live as a widow/widower?
- Is my sense of my physical self such that predictable physical
  changes with age can be absorbed into a healthy self-esteem?

- Do my attitudes toward the opposite sex preclude learning opposite gender skills that will be needed or useful in later years?
- What can I learn from older family members (and other older adults) about what I do and do not want as part of my own late life years?

These questions occur in a context of understanding the adult life span to be (on the average) six or seven decades, of which four or so will be spent working and perhaps two decades will be spent raising a family. Two or more decades will be spent in either the postretirement, empty-nest marriage or the widowed lifestyle that comprises old age. Rather than ignoring this future until the last moment, it can be planned for throughout adulthood. Rather than defining optimal adult life as early or middle adulthood, the emerging model of maturity described here can be taken seriously and cultivated.

In my own life so far, the impact of thinking about the adult life span in these terms has been mixed. The realization of how long we live as adults has brought the relief of knowing that there is time to achieve goals and to work out personal problems. On the positive side, anticipating my own future has led me to place a great value on fatherhood. I do not want to join the ranks of men who discover only in their young-old years that they missed parenthood. On the negative side, I am aware that my focus on career and work does not prepare me well for life after retirement.

In working with clients, the prospective view prompts me to encourage them to think about whether there are unresolved issues with relatives who have life-threatening illnesses or who are among the old-old. Clients caring for frail spouses are encouraged to anticipate widowhood. Clients who are trying to work out a postretirement life-style are encouraged to plan for a couple of decades.

The maturity-specific challenge model for work with older adults, and the prospective view of the life span as outlined in this chapter, can challenge therapists to prepare themselves to confront directly the major problems of the final third of life. The concept of lifelong maturation reminds us of the strengths and the experience that older clients bring to the task of working out solutions to these problems. A clear image of positive maturity in late life will ensure that those clients who have aged without maturing

		Young		Post-Retirement
Childhood⟶	Adolescence⟶	Adulthood⟶	Adulthood⟶	Life
12 yrs	8 yrs	10 yrs	30 yrs	20 to 30 yrs

Figure 2. The Human Life Span

will be recognized as having unfinished developmental tasks to complete in therapy. These concepts can guide psychotherapy with older adults beyond supportive therapy with kindly elders in a second childhood of dependency and frailty and into the challenging work of confronting serious problems with a client who may be more mature than his or her therapist.

References

Abraham, K. (1919/1977). The applicability of psychoanalytic treatment to patients at an advanced age. In S. Steury & M. L. Blank (Eds.), *Readings in psychotherapy with older people* (pp. 18-20). Washington, DC: Department of Health, Education, and Welfare.

Baltes, P. B., & Baltes, M. M. (1990). Psychological perspectives on successful aging: The model of selective optimization with compensation. In P. B. Baltes & M. M. Baltes (Eds.), *Successful aging: A psychological model* (pp. 1-34). Cambridge, MA: Cambridge University Press.

Bandura, A. (1982). Self-efficacy mechanism in human agency. *American Psychologist, 37*, 122-147.

Begnston, V. L., Reedy, M. N., & Gordon, C. (1985). Aging and self-conceptions: Personality processes and social contexts. In J. E. Birren & K. W. Schaie (Eds.), *Handbook of the psychology of aging* (2nd ed.) (pp. 544-593). New York: Van Nostrand Reinhold.

Bennet, R. (1983). The socially isolated elderly. In M. K. Aronson, R. Bennet, & B. J. Gurland (Eds.), *The acting-out elderly* (pp. 45-54). New York: Haworth.

Berezin, M. (1963). Some intrapsychic aspects of aging. In N. E. Zinsberg & I. Kaufman (Eds.), *Normal psychology of the aging process*. New York: International Universities Press.

Birren, J. E., & Deutchman, D. E. (1990). *Guiding autobiography group for older adults: Exploring the future of life*. Baltimore, MD: Johns Hopkins University Press.

Bornstein, R., & Smircina, M. T. (1982). The status of empirical support for the hypothesis of increased variability in aging populations. *The Gerontologist, 22*, 258-260.

Botwinick, J. (1984). *Aging and behavior* (3rd ed.). New York: Springer.

Breytspraak, L. M. (1984). *The development of self in later life*. Boston: Little, Brown.

Brown, F. H. (1988). The impact of death and serious illness on the family life cycle. In B. Carter & M. McGoldrick (Eds.), *The changing family life cycle* (pp. 457-482). New York: Gardner Press.

Bumagin, V. E., & Hirn, K. F. (1990). *Helping the aging family*. Glenview, IL: Scott, Foresman.

Butler, R. N., & Lewis, M. I. (1982). *Aging and mental health*. St. Louis: C. V. Mosby.

Carter, B., & McGoldrick, M. (Eds.). (1988). *The changing family life cycle.* New York: Gardner Press.

Cohen, C. I. (1987). Elderly schizophrenics and paranoiacs living in single-room-occupancy hotels. In N. E. Miller & G. D. Cohen (Eds.), *Schizophrenia and aging* (pp. 206-213). New York: Guilford.

Cohen, G. D. (1987). Psychotherapeutic approaches to schizophrenia in later life. In N. E. Miller & G. D. Cohen (Eds.), *Schizophrenia and aging* (pp. 287-298). New York: Guilford.

Cohler, B. J., & Ferrono, C. L. (1987). Schizophrenia and the adult life-course. In N. E. Miller & G. D. Cohen (Eds.), *Schizophrenia and aging* (pp. 189-199). New York: Guilford.

Costa, P. T., & McCrae, R. R. (1985). Hypochondriasis, neuroticism, and aging: When are somatic complaints unfounded? *American Psychologist, 40,* 19-28.

Costa, P. T., McCrae, R. R., & Arenberg, D. (1983). Recent longitudinal research on personality and aging. In K. W. Schaie (Ed.), *Longitudinal studies of adult psychological development.* New York: Guilford.

Costa, P. T., Zonderman, A. B., McCrae, R. R., Cornoni-Huntley, J., Locke, B. Z., & Barbano, H. E. (1987). Longitudinal analysis of psychological well-being in a national sample: Stability of mean levels. *Journal of Gerontology, 42,* 50-56.

Craik, F.I.M., & Trehub, S. (1982). *Aging and cognitive processes.* New York: Plenum.

de Rivera, J. (1984). Development and the full range of emotional expression. In C. Z. Malatesta & C. E. Izard (Eds.), *Emotion in adult development* (pp. 45-63). Beverly Hills, CA: Sage.

Erickson, M. H. (1980). *Collected papers of Milton H. Erickson on hypnosis.* Ernest L. Rossi (Ed.). NY: Halstead.

Erikson, E. H. (1968). *Identity: Youth and crisis.* New York: Norton.

Ewing, C. P. (1978). *Crisis intervention as psychotherapy.* New York: Oxford University Press.

Felton, B. J., & Revenson, T. (1987). Age differences in coping with chronic illness. *Psychology and Aging, 2,* 164-170.

Finch, C. E., & Morgan, D. (1987). Aging and schizophrenia: A hypothesis relating asynchrony in neural aging processes to the manifestations of schizophrenia and other neurologic diseases with age. In N. E. Miller & G. D. Cohen (Eds.), *Schizophrenia and aging* (pp. 97-108). New York: Guilford.

Folkman, S., Lazarus, R. S., Pimley, S., & Novacek, J. (1987). Age differences in stress and coping processes. *Psychology and Aging, 2,* 171-184.

Folstein, M. F., Folstein, S. E., & McHugh, P. R. (1975). "Mini-Mental state": A practical method for grading the cognitive state of patients for the clinician. *Journal of Psychiatric Research, 12,* 189-198.

Frankfather, D. (1977). *The aged in the community.* New York: Praeger.

Gatz, M., & Hurwicz, M. (1990). Are older people more depressed? Cross-sectional data on Center for Epidemiological Studies depression scale factors. *Psychology and Aging, 5,* 284-290.

Gendlin, E. (1978). *Focusing.* New York: Everest House.

Genevay, B., & Katz, R. S. (1990). *Countertransference and older clients.* Newbury Park, CA: Sage.

Gitelson, M. (1948). The emotional problems of elderly people. *Geriatrics, 3,* 135-150.

Goldfried, M. R., & Davison, G. (1976). *Clinical behavior theory.* New York: Holt.

Goldstein, A. P. (1973). *Structured learning therapy: Toward a therapy for the poor.* New York: Academic Press.

Gottman, J., Notarius, C., Gonzo, J., & Markman, H. (1976). *A couple's guide to communication.* Champaign, IL: Research Press.

Gutmann, D. (1987). *Reclaimed powers: Toward a new psychology of men and women in later life.* New York: Basic Books.

Gynther, M. D. (1979). Aging and personality. In J. N. Butcher (Ed.), *New developments in the use of the MMPI* (pp. 39-68). Minneapolis: University of Minnesota Press.

Haan, N., Millsap, R., & Hartka, E. (1986). As time goes by: Change and stability in personality over fifty years. *Psychology and Aging, 1*(3), 220-232.

Hall, C. M. (1981). *The Bowen family theory and its uses.* New York: Jason Aronson.

Jung, C. J. (1933). *Modern man in search of a soul.* New York: Harcourt Brace & World.

Kelly, G. A. (1955). *The psychology of personal constructs.* New York: Norton.

Knight, B. G. (1983). Assessing a mobile outreach team. In M. A. Smyer & M. Gatz (Eds.), *Mental health and aging: Programs and evaluations.* Beverly Hills, CA: Sage.

Knight, B. G. (1986). *Psychotherapy with older adults.* Beverly Hills, CA: Sage.

Knight, B. G. (1988). Factors influencing therapist-rated change in older adults. *Journal of Gerontology, 43,* 111-112.

Knight, B. G. (1989). *Outreach with the elderly: Community education, assessment, and therapy.* New York: New York University Press.

Kübler-Ross, E. (1969). *On death and dying.* New York: Macmillan.

Labouvie-Vief, G., DeVoe, M., & Bulka, D. (1989). Speaking about feelings: Conceptions of emotion across the life span. *Psychology and Aging, 4*(4), 425-437.

Lamb, H. R. (1987). Predisposition to schizophrenia: Breakdown or adaptation in later life. In N. E. Miller & G. D. Cohen (Eds.), *Schizophrenia and aging* (pp. 200-205). New York: Guilford Press.

Lehman, D. R., Ellard, J. H., & Wortman, C. B. (1986). Social support for the bereaved: Recipients' and providers' perspectives on what is helpful. *Journal of Personality and Social Psychology, 54,* 438-446.

Lewinsohn, P. M., & MacPhillamy, D. J. (1974). The relationship between age and engagement in pleasant activities. *Journal of Gerontology, 29,* 290-294.

Lewinsohn, P. M., Munoz, R. F., Youngren, M. A., & Zeiss, A. M. (1978). *Control your depression.* Englewood Cliffs, NJ: Prentice-Hall.

Light, E., & Lebowitz, B. (1990). *Alzheimer's disease treatment and family stress.* Washington, DC: Hemisphere.

Light, L. L. (1990). Interactions between memory and language in old age. In J. E. Birren & K. W. Schaie (Eds.), *Handbook of the psychology of aging* (3rd ed.) (pp. 275-290). New York: Academic Press.

Longino, C. F., & Kant, C. S. (1982). Explicating activity theory: A formal replication. *Journal of Gerontology, 37,* 713-722.

Lorion, R. P. (1978). Research on psychotherapy and behavior change with the disadvantaged. In S. L. Garfield & A. E. Bergin (Eds.), *Handbook of psychotherapy and behavior change* (pp. 903-938). New York: John Wiley.

Mace, N., & Rabins, P. (1982). *The 36 hour day.* Baltimore, MD: Johns Hopkins University Press.

MacKinnon, R. A., & Michaels, R. (1971). *The psychiatric interview in clinical practice.* Philadelphia: W. B. Saunders.

Malatesta, C. Z., & Izard, C. E. (1984). The facial expression of emotion: Young, middle-aged, and older adult expressions. In C. Z. Malatesta & C. E. Izard (Eds.), *Emotion in adult development* (pp. 253-273). Beverly Hills, CA: Sage.

Margolin, G. (1982). Ethical and legal considerations in marital and family therapy. *American Psychologist, 37*, 788-801.

Maslow, A. H. (1970). *Motivation and personality* (2nd ed.). New York: Harper & Row.

Masters, W. H., & Johnson, V. E. (1970). *Human sexual inadequacy*. Boston: Little, Brown.

McCrae, R. R., & Costa, P. T. (1984). *Emerging lives, enduring dispositions: Personality in adulthood*. Boston: Little, Brown.

McMurtry, L. (1985). *Lonesome dove*. New York: Simon & Schuster.

Miller, N. E., & Cohen, G. D. (Eds.). (1987). *Schizophrenia and aging*. New York: Guilford.

Myers, J. K., & Associates. (1984). Six month prevalence of psychiatric disorders in three communities. *Archives of General Psychiatry, 41*, 959-967.

Neugarten, B. L. (1977). Personality and aging. In J. E. Birren & K. W. Schaie (Eds.), *Handbook of the psychology of aging*. New York: Van Nostrand Reinhold.

Neugarten, B. L., & Hagestad, G. O. (1976). Age and the life course. In R. H. Binstock & E. Shanas (Eds.), *Handbook of aging and the social sciences*. New York: Van Nostrand Reinhold.

Niederehe, G., & Rusin, M. J. (1987). Schizophrenia and aging: Information processing patterns. In N. E. Miller & G. D. Cohen (Eds.), *Schizophrenia and aging* (pp. 162-179). New York: Guilford.

Pearlin, L., Turner, H., & Semple, S. (1989). Coping in mediation of caregiver stress. In E. Light & B. Lebowitz (Eds.), *Alzheimer's disease treatment and family stress*. Washington, DC: Hemisphere.

Pearlin, L. I., Mullan, J. T., Semple, S. J., & Skaff, M. M. (1990). Caregiving and the stress process: An overview of concepts and their measures. *The Gerontologist, 30*, 583-594.

Peters-Golden, H. (1982). Breast cancer: Varied perceptions of social support in the illness experience. *Social Science and Medicine, 16*, 483-491.

Polster, E., & Polster, M. (1973). *Gestalt therapy integrated*. New York: Vintage.

Poon, L. W. (1985). Differences in human memory with aging: Nature, causes, and clinical implications. In J. E. Birren & K. W. Schaie (Eds.), *Handbook of the psychology of aging* (2nd ed.) (pp. 427-462). New York: Van Nostrand Reinhold.

Rando, T. A. (1984). *Grief, dying, and death*. Champaign, IL: Research Press.

Rechtschaffen, A. (1959). Psychotherapy with geriatric patients: A review of the literature. *Journal of Gerontology, 14*, 73-84.

Reisberg, B., Shulman, E., Ferris, S. H., de Leon, M. J., & Geibel, V. (1983). Clinical assessments of age-associated cognitive decline and primary degenerative dementia: Prognostic concomitants. *Psychopharmacology Bulletin, 19*, 734-739.

Rodin, J., & Salovey, P. (1989). Health psychology. *Annual Review of Psychology, 40*, 533-579.

Rook, K. S. (1984). The negative side of social interaction: Impact on psychological well-being. *Journal of Personality and Social Psychology, 46*, 1097-1108.

Roth, M. (1987). Late paraphrenia: Phenomenology and etiological factors and their bearing upon problems of the schizophrenic family of disorders. In N. E. Miller & G. D. Cohen (Eds.), *Schizophrenia and aging* (pp. 217-234). New York: Guilford.

Rybash, J. M., Hoyer, W. J., & Roodin, P. A. (1986). *Adult cognition and aging.* Elmsford, NY: Pergamon.

Salthouse, T. A. (1985). Speed of behavior and its implications for cognition. In J. E. Birren & K. W. Schaie (Eds.), *Handbook of the psychology of aging* (2nd ed.) (pp. 400-426). New York: Van Nostrand Reinhold.

Schaie, K. W. (Ed.). (1983). *Longitudinal studies of adult psychological development.* New York: Guilford.

Schulz, R. (1982). Emotionality and aging: A theoretical and empirical analysis. *Journal of Gerontology, 37,* 42-51.

Shanas, E. (1979). Social myth as hypothesis: The case of the family relations of old people. *The Gerontologist, 19,* 3-9.

Sherman, E. (1981). *Counseling the aging.* New York: Free Press.

Siegler, I. C. (1983). Psychological aspects of the Duke Longitudinal Studies. In K. W. Schaie (Ed.), *Longitudinal studies of adult psychological development* (pp. 136-190). New York: Guilford.

Simon, R. M. (1988). Family life cycle issues in the therapy system. In B. Carter & M. McGoldrick (Eds.), *The changing family life cycle* (pp. 108-117). New York: Gardner Press.

Singer, J. L. (1974). *Imagery and daydream methods in psychotherapy and behavior modification.* New York: Academic Press.

Tinsley, H. E. A., Teaff, J. D., Colbs, S. L., & Kaufman, N. (1985). A system of classifying leisure activities in terms of the psychological benefits of participation reported by older persons. *Journal of Gerontology, 40,* 172-178.

Walsh, F. (1988). The family in later life. In B. Carter & M. McGoldrick (Eds.), *The changing family life cycle.* New York: Gardner Press.

Ward, R. A., Sherman, S. R., & LaGary, M. (1984). Subjective network assessment and subjective well-being. *Journal of Gerontology, 39,* 93-101.

Wollert, R. W., Knight, B. G., & Levy, L. H. (1980). MTC: A collaborative model for professionals and self-help groups. *Professional Psychology, 11,* 130-138.

Woodruff, D. S. (1985). Arousal, sleep, and aging. In J. E. Birren & K. W. Schaie (Eds.), *Handbook of the psychology of aging* (2nd ed.) (pp. 261-295). New York: Van Nostrand Reinhold.

Woodruff, D. S., & Birren, J. E. (1972). Age changes and cohort differences in personality. *Developmental Psychology, 6,* 252-259.

Worden, W. (1982). *Grief counseling and grief therapy.* New York: Springer.

Zarit, S. H. (1980). *Aging and mental disorders.* New York: Free Press.

Zarit, S. H., Orr, N., & Zarit, J. (1985). *Hidden victims of Alzheimer's disease: Families under stress.* New York: New York University Press.

About the Author

Bob G. Knight, Ph.D., is the Merle H. Bensinger Associate Professor of Gerontology and Psychology at the Andrus Gerontology Center, University of Southern California. In that position, he serves as director of the Andrus Older Adult Center and the Los Angeles Caregiver Resource Center. He has published extensively in mental health and aging, including *Psychotherapy with Older Adults* (Sage, 1986) and *Outreach with the Elderly* (NYU Press, 1989).